Introduction

Safety is the first concern when out on the sea. This applies not only to the equipment and gear, but it is also essential as it relates to the medical equipment and the level of training of all those who go boating or sailing.

The stakes are high, because in the case of illness or accident, medical assistance might be hard to get—it might even be impossible. While the "first aid" on land might only last for a few minutes until the arrival of paramedics, this first aid might be the only aid for hours, or days, when onboard a seagoing vessel and, in the case of a lack of treatment options, even minor accidents, such as burns or injuries, can cause an unwanted interruption of the trip. Serious illness or major accidents can result in a catastrophe.

First aid training and knowledge should be a given for everyone who is going to sea. Because of the challenging situation and special circumstances—far from quick help—a course about "medicine on board" is not only strongly recommended, but also a very useful addition.

The intent of this book is to provide a quick and handy overview for the medical layperson: what are my options regarding the most common medical problems at sea? How can I collect relevant information about a sick or injured person? Such information is valuable for first aid help as well as for help over the radio, because it may facilitate decisions about the treatment strategy and hence save lives under extreme circumstances.

I wish you a good and safe trip without unforeseen events. Should there be an emergency, I hope this book helps you to do the right thing at the right time.

Fabian Steffen,
April 2014

Please keep the following in mind:
- You are solely responsible for all of your actions.
- You and any other person aboard have the duty to help within your capabilities.
- In case of available professional help, limit yourself to the immediate and necessary actions.
- If there is no medical help available, you may have to act independently.
- Make sure you procure medical help early on.
- Take part in first aid courses on a regular basis. This way you will not hesitate to act during an emergency.

Before the Trip

Before taking a journey out to sea, it is important to be well-prepared. This includes preventive checkups, vaccinations, procuring the necessary medical equipment and medicine, as well as important paperwork and forms.

> **TIP** You can find the forms on the Internet at **www.seadoc.de.** Print them out before the trip. These forms are available in both English and German. You can find a short version of these forms in the Appendix on Page 82.
>
> ### Medical Information
> Each passenger should provide information about his or her medical condition before a trip or journey. Such medical information may be important in case of an emergency.
>
> ### Checkup
> Always get a check-up prior to a trip. Fill in the results.
>
> ### Radio-assisted Consultation
> This guide prepares you for reporting a medical emergency via radio transmission and, if needed, a consultation.
>
> ### Protocol
> Medical situations change quickly – in order to stay on top of the situation, regular updates are important.

To Do List — Medical Preparations Before Journeying Out to Sea

- Optimize physical fitness
- See your doctor: Medical checkup, treat and stabilize underlying conditions, determine drug requirements (regular medication, emergency, and other medication and drugs), consult about defibrillators (if appropriate for use onboard, risk factors, etc., see page 11)
- See your doctor (or expert for tropical diseases): Check vaccination status (refresh standard vaccinations, check for additional prevention)
- If applicable, see a pediatrician: Check child's medication and vaccination dates during the trip
- Purchase and store medicine, drugs, and medical equipment (Pages 68-70)
- Refresh first aid knowledge, preferably with emphasis on treatments onboard a seagoing vessel (Page 82)
- Print-out important forms and bring then with you
- Annotate emergency contact numbers and practice VHF communication with all participants (Page 5)

Bring it with you — Medical Equipment for the Journey

Common medical problems on board
- **Small and large wounds**
- **Burn wounds**
- **Injuries to limbs:** e.g. bruise, sprain, bone fracture (rare)
  Life-threatening situations are rare, but they are always dramatic. In order to be able to deal with them, you need to have the proper equipment and medication or drugs.

Equipment and Medication
- **Wounds:** Cleaning (swabs, antiseptic, tools like scissors, tweezers, scalpel) and care (wound dressings, band aids, gauze bandages; Page 64)
- **Burn wounds:** Materials to avoid infection and scar formation (Page 51)
- **Injuries of the limbs:** Cooling materials and stabilization (immobilizing bandages, splint, triangular scarf or bandage; Page 55)
- **Life-threatening situations:** Emergency blankets against hypothermia, tube to keep respiratory passages open, ventilation barrier for mouth-to-mouth resuscitation (Page 6), defibrillator if possible
- **Medicines and drugs:** Suggestions starting on Page 67

Other Valuable Items to Have
- Thermometer, examination gloves, automatic blood pressure monitor, emergency kit for teeth, eye rinse kit
- For sea journeys to areas with doubtful sanitation standards: Materials for sterilization in clinics and medical practices (e.g. syringes and hypodermic needles/cannules)
- Additionally, for experienced persons: Bag valve mask, equipment to provide drugs or liquid intravenously such as into a muscle or a blood vessel (starting on Page 79)

> **IMPORTANT**
>
> The equipment must be adequate for the maritime environment, of good quality, and contained in waterproof storage. The volume should correspond to the number of people aboard (starting on Page 67).

The Emergency Call

The emergency call's purpose is to notify professional assistance. At sea, the coordination of all emergencies is handled by United States Coast Guard Rescue Coordination Centers (RCC). When contacting them, be sure to have the following information on hand:

- **Medical and general information form (to be filled out by each passenger ahead of the journey; these forms are available at www.seadoc.de in both English and German):**
  - Age, weight, height, name and contact details of relatives and family physician, blood pressure and pulse at rest, pre-existing conditions, surgeries, drugs and their place of storage, allergies
- **Essential basic information for radio-assisted medical help:**
  - Who is calling, position, nearest port
  - Patient's name, sex, age, pre-existing conditions, drugs
  - Vital parameters: Consciousness, respiration, circulation
  - Main problem: When did it begin, cause, suspected diagnosis
  - In case of accident: Affected area, description
- **Additional information:**
  - Examine the patient thoroughly and annotate the findings (examination form)
  - Check the medication and drugs available on board

> ⚠ The emergency call can be done via telephone or VHF radio. However, please note that even in these modern technology times, a cell phone connection at sea is unreliable. In case of an emergency, do not waste time trying to get a signal; instead, focus on to establishing contact via VHF radio. Satellite telephones provide connections even when far away from land, e.g. on the Atlantic Ocean. Be sure to get a list of contact numbers before the journey.

Emergency call via VHF:

If there is a digital VHF radio onboard, the first step is to make an automatic emergency call using channel 70 (DSC–Digital Selective Calling). Next, make a VHF call using channel 16 to the closest USCG RCC of the corresponding region. Make sure you familiarize yourself with the procedure before starting your journey or trip!

Emergency call via Telephone

Information from the website of the United States Coast Guard Search & Rescue; information last modified December 4, 2013.

- **Atlantic Area SAR Coordinator, Portsmouth, Virginia, 757-398-6700:** Overall responsibility for areas covered by RCC Boston, Norfolk, Miami, San Juan, New Orleans, and Cleveland, plus a portion of the North Atlantic Ocean out to 40 degrees west longitude
- **RCC Boston, Boston, Massachusetts, 617-223-8555:** New England down to and including a portion of Northern New Jersey, plus the U.S. waters of Lake Champlain
- **RCC Norfolk, Portsmouth, Virginia, 757-398-6231:** Mid-Atlantic states including the majority of New Jersey down to the North Carolina-South Carolina border
- **RCC Miami, Miami, Florida, 305-415-6800:** Southeast states from the South Carolina-North Carolina border around to the eastern end of the Florida panhandle, plus a large portion of the Caribbean Sea.
- **RSC San Juan (sub-center of RCC Miami), San Juan, Puerto Rico, 787-289-2042:** Southeast portion of the Caribbean Sea
- **RCC New Orleans, New Orleans, Louisiana, 504-589-6225:** Southern states from the Florida panhandle to the U.S.-Mexico border in Texas and the inland rivers including the Mississippi, Missouri, Ohio, and tributaries
- **RCC Cleveland, Cleveland, Ohio, 216-902-6117:** U.S. waters of the Great Lakes, their connecting rivers, and tributaries
- **Pacific SAR Coordinator, Alameda, California, 510-437-3700:** Overall responsibility for areas covered by RCC Alameda, Seattle, Honolulu, and Juneau
- **RCC Alameda, Alameda, California, 510-437-3700:** California and Eastern Pacific Ocean waters assigned by international convention off the Coast of Mexico
- **RCC Seattle, Seattle, Washington, 206-220-7001:** Oregon and Washington
- **RCC Honolulu (operated as JRCC with DOD), Honolulu, Hawaii, 808-535-3333:** Hawaii, U.S. Pacific Islands, and the waters of Central Pacific Ocean assigned by the international convention, extending from as far as 6 degrees south to 40 degrees north latitude and as far as 110 west to 130 east longitude
- **Sector Guam (coordinates SAR under RCC Honolulu), SectorGuam, 671-355-4824:** Guam and other U.S. territories in the far western Pacific Ocean
- **RCC Juneau, Juneau, Alaska, 907-463-2000:** Alaska and the U.S. waters in North Pacific Ocean, Bering Sea, and Arctic Ocean

3 x Mayday	1 x MMSI number
"This is . . ."	Position and time (UTC) (see [2] below)
3 x name of vessel	Message: information regarding
1 x Call sign	• type of emergency
1 x MMSI number (see [1] below)	• required help
1 x Mayday	(e.g. "we need urgent medical help!")
1 x Name of vessel	• additional information
1 x Call sign	Over

Usually, a confirmation is received within 15 seconds via the RCC or another vessel.

(1) MMSI: Personal identification number assigned with the radio frequency

Life-threatening Situations

In life-threatening situations, vital signs can be disturbed or non-existent. These situations require immediate action and professional help as soon as possible.

> **Vital Parameters**
> ↘ Consciousness ↘ Respiration ↘ Circulation

Causes for Life-threatening Situations
1. Unconsciousness
2. Bleeding profusely
3. Major breathing difficulty
4. Impaired consciousness with self-endangerment

> **IMPORTANT**
>
> With every assistance ...
> ↘ Avoid putting yourself in danger
> ↘ Respect your own safety
> ↘ Act calmly
> ↘ Call for help immediately or make emergency call (or have someone make the call for you)

What to do in Life-threatening Situations?
1. **First Step:** Remove injured person from the source of danger (e.g. fire, loose items); utilize rescue grip (figure 1) or secure with life belt
2. **Second Step:** Check vital signs... Does the patient respond? Is he breathing? (Page 9, Reanimation)
3. **Third Step:** Get help
   ↘ At Port: Shout for help; make emergency call (PROVIDE NUMBERS)
   ↘ At Sea: Make emergency call (Page 5)

> **IMPORTANT**
>
> Do not waste time; begin assistance immediately (Page 7).

The Rescue Grip
↘ Used to transport or move unconscious persons in case of immediate threat to life (fire, going overboard)
↘ Apply immediately...even prior to checking vital signs!

How to do the Rescue Grip
- Raise the patient's upper body.
- Grab one of the patient's lower arms through both armpits.
- Raise the patient and remove him from the danger zone.

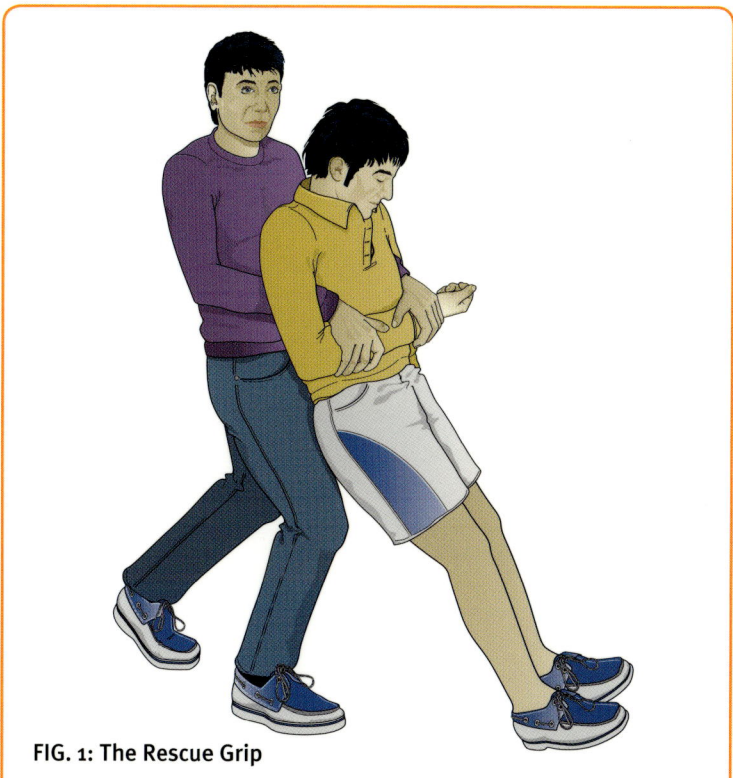

FIG. 1: The Rescue Grip

Life-threatening Situations – Unconsciousness

Causes
- Accident involving the head (Page 59)
- Cardiac arrest, cardiac arrhythmia (Page 40)
- Shock (Page 41)
- Sickness and poisoning (starting at Page 34)
- Hypothermia (Page 49)
- Sunstroke (Page 50)

How to recognize?
- **Immediately:** Sudden collapse without defensive movement or reflex in case of cardiac arrest, cardiac irregularity, cramp or stroke
- **Delayed:** In case of poisoning, hypothermia, or sunstroke

What can happen?
- Death by unrecognized absence of breathing or cardiac arrest
- Major brain damage or death if reanimation procedures are delayed

> **TIP** Every second counts! It's important to regularly check the patient's breathing and heartbeat while providing help.

What to do?
Check vital parameters: consciousness, breathing, heartbeat (Page 9)
- Unconscious, with breathing and heartbeat: stable lateral position (figure 3, page 8), possibly breathing tube (figure 2)
- Unconsciousness and respiratory arrest with heartbeat: artificial respiration (figure 4, page 10), possibly breathing tube (figure 2)
- Unconsciousness, respiratory and cardiac arrest: resuscitation (Page 9)

Artificial Respiration
A breathing tube …
- is designed to keep the airways clear
- reduces the risk of asphyxiation for patients with impaired consciousness
- can be inserted before and during the stable lateral position
- can facilitate artificial respiration
- provides an additional protection against asphyxiation while in a stable lateral position
- is available for all body sizes; suggested sizes: 5/16" (8mm) diameter for larger, 1/4" (7mm) diameter for smaller adults

How to do – Insert Breathing Tube
- Moisten tube
- Insert with a rotating motion and only little pressure up to the ring at the end of the tube into one of the unconscious patient's nostrils (figure 2)

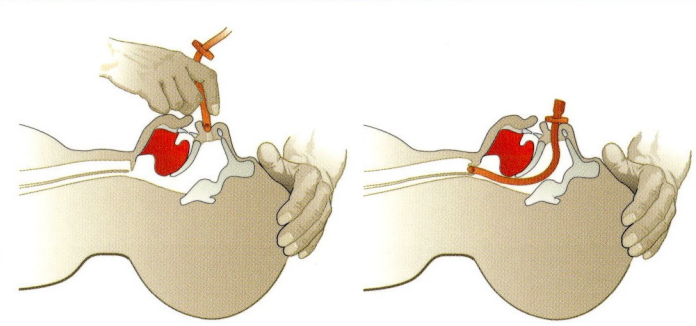

Figure 2: Insert breathing tube

> ⚠ Breathing tubes can lead to bruises inside the mouth and throat areas, so do not use force! Check regularly that the unconscious person is still breathing. If not, artificial respiration must be given.

The Stable Lateral Position
- Minimizes the risk of asphyxiation
- Must only be used if the patient is breathing
- Breathing must be controlled regularly

How to Perform the Stable Lateral Position

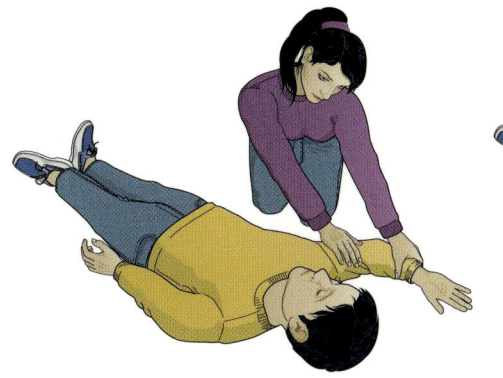

1 Bend one arm

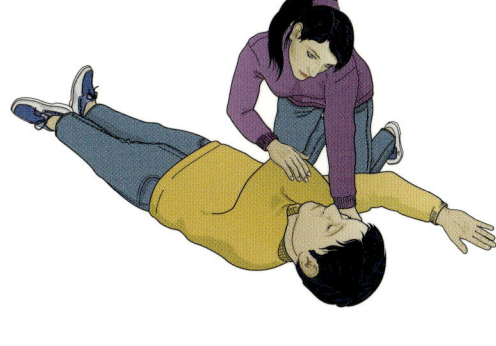

2 Pull the elbow of the other arm over the chest; place your hand on the cheek of the opposite side

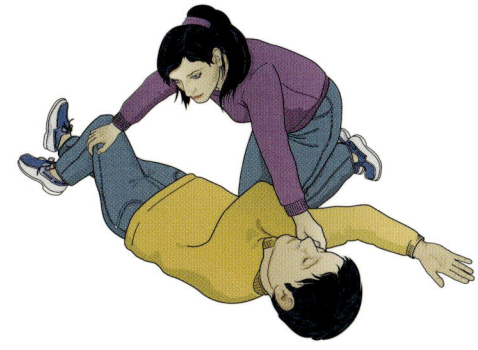

3 Turn the body towards the bent arm (see 1); position the upper leg as shown to stabilize

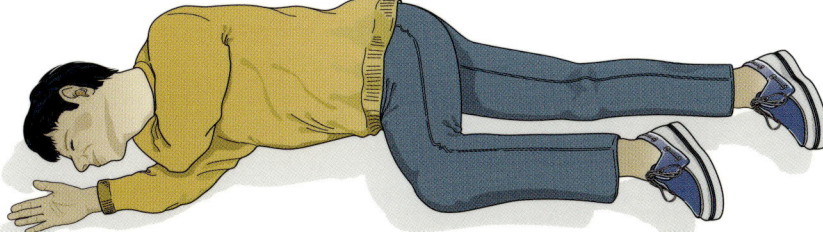

Figure 3: The Stable Lateral Position

Life-threatening Situations – Unconsciousness

Resuscitating an Unconscious Person

⬊ **Check vital signs and open breathing passages:** They can be obstructed by the tongue.
⬊ **Cardiac massage:** Cardiac arrest causes the blood flow to stop. Organ damage happens quickly, particularly to the brain.
⬊ **Resuscitate:** It provides the blood in the lungs with oxygen.

Control is important: The chest must clearly be moving. It is best to remove clothing (scissors, rip apart).

Other measures
⬊ Apply defibrillator (Page 11)
⬊ Assist artificial respiration with a breathing tube (Page 7)

When to end resuscitation efforts
Resuscitation efforts should only be ended when …
⬊ Consciousness and breathing return
⬊ Professional help arrives
⬊ Signs of certain death appear
⬊ The rescuers are exhausted

How to Resuscitate a Person

①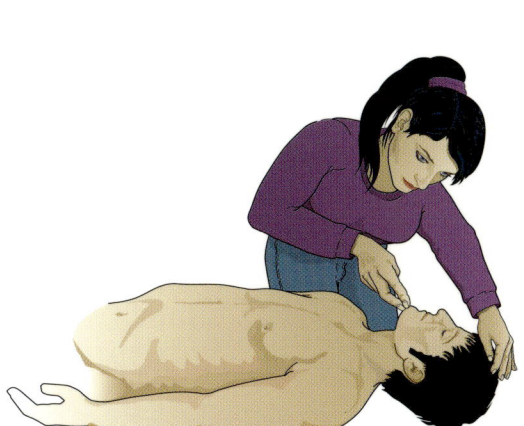

②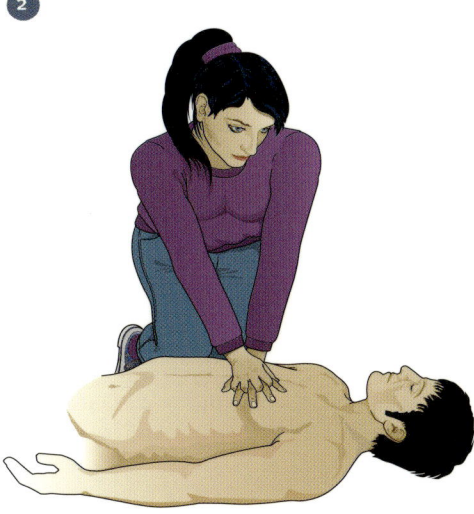

③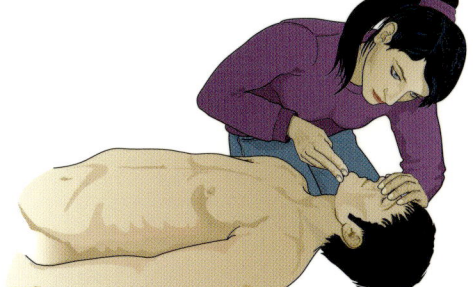

Figure 4: Resuscitation

① Check vital signs and open breathing passages

Check vital signs
- **Consciousness:** Address with a loud voice, shake, pinch
- **Breathing:** Observe upper body (Page 24)
- **Heartbeat:** Check pulse (not recommended for novices!)

No breathing or hesitating breathing? Then:
Open breathing passages
- Raise chin at the lower jaw
- Slightly stretch the neck
- Remove obstacles (e.g. food, artificial denture)

Total Time: No more than 10 seconds!

② Cardiac massage (30 x)
- The pressure point is around the middle of the sternum.
- Press with the palm **30 x with at least a frequency of 100 per minute and a pressure depth of 2 inches** (5cm).
- Cardiac massage is exhausting, so change position every 3-5 minutes.
- Keep pauses as short as possible.

③ Artificial respiration (2 x)
- Place head as shown in Step 1.
- **Resuscitate 2 x in no more than 5 seconds** (mouth-to-mouth or mouth-to-nose).
- Keep breathing passages open using a breathing tube (see figure 2, page 7).

④ Continue with 2 and 3 alternating:
30 x cardiac massage and 2 x resuscitation.

Life-threatening Situations – Unconsciousness

Resuscitation with Defibrillator
Defibrillators are used to treat ventricular fibrillation. Ventricular fibrillation is the uncoordinated activity (fibrillation) of the heart muscle, leading to an immediate cardiac arrest. Fibrillation can only be stopped utilizing so-called defibrillation: the heart muscle activity is supposed to be coordinated again via an electric shock.

> ⚠️ Risk factors for ventricular fibrillation are restrictions of the coronary vessels and known cardiac arrhythmias. Other factors include certain age groups, obesity, and smoking. Ask your family physician whether you are part of a high-risk group.

Using it onboard a sea-going vessel
The use of a defibrillator onboard a ship or other sea-going vessel is safe; modern equipment automatically determines the need for defibrillation. Even novices can use it and it is recommended. However, not all types of equipment are apt for their use onboard.

> **IMPORTANT**
>
> Defibrillation is an addition to other measures of resuscitation, such as cardiac massage and artificial respiration, not a replacement.

Application by one helper
- If a defibrillator is readily available and unconsciousness has been detected: Apply the defibrillator immediately.
- Turn on the equipment and follow the voice commands; an automatic analysis of the cardiac rhythm is performed.
- If recommended, initiate defibrillation.

Application by more than one helper
- One or more helpers initiate resuscitation.
- Another helper gets the defibrillator, connects it to the patient, and turns it on.

How to Use the Defibrillator
- Remove clothing from upper body: Rip up clothing or cut it up (even expensive clothes!).
- If necessary, towel off skin.
- Turn on defibrillator and follow instructions.
- If the defibrillator recommends a shock or if it is performed automatically: Do not touch the patient!
- Continue with the resuscitation efforts immediately after the shock.
- If no shock is recommended or if the automatic defibrillator does not function, resume resuscitation efforts immediately.

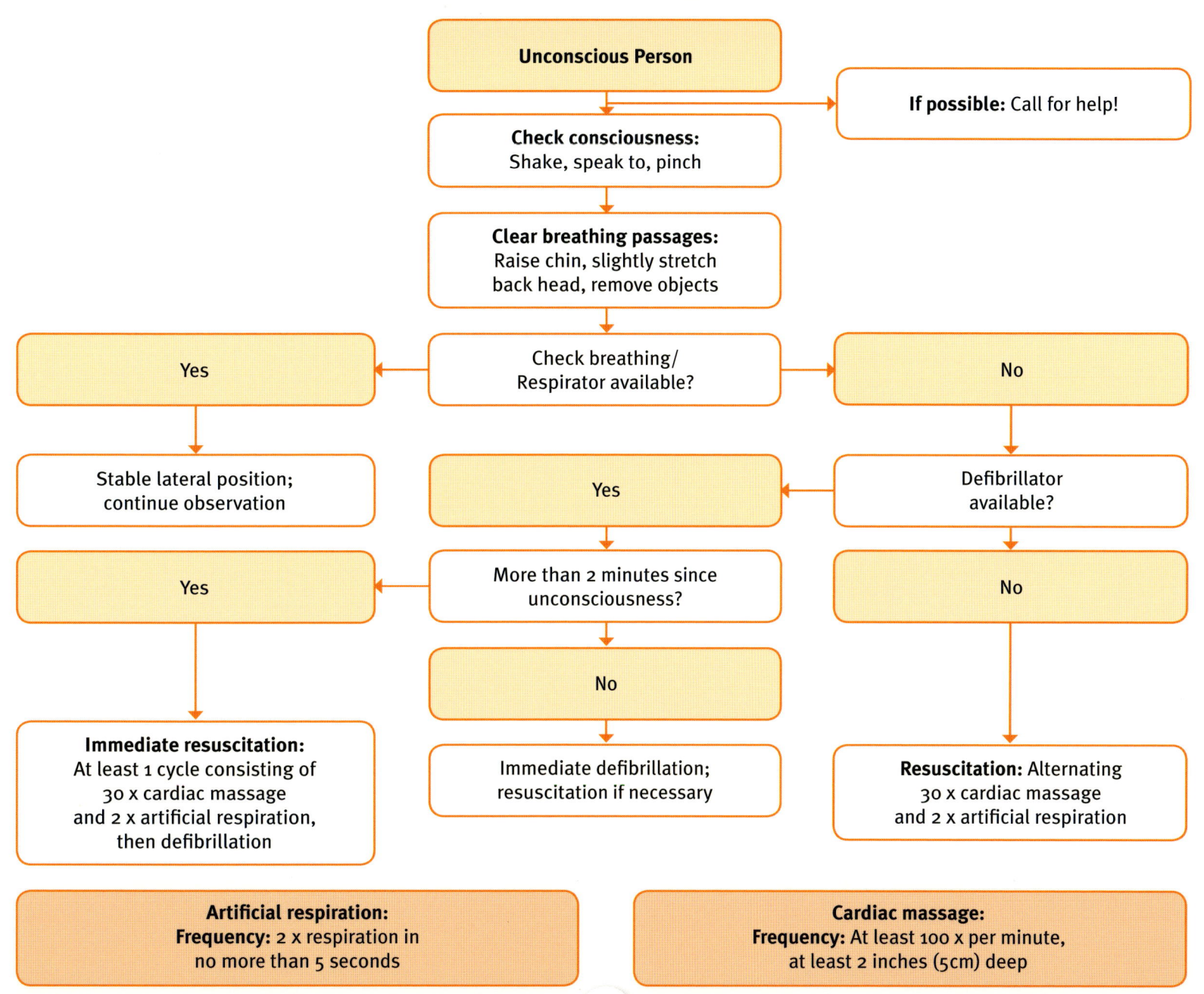

Life-threatening Situations – Massive Bleeding

Causes
- Large wound
- Wounds occurring after prior ingestion of anticoagulant drugs (such as Aspirin®, Marcumar®, Plavix®)

How to recognize
- Visible exterior bleeding
- Invisible interior bleeding (e.g. damage of organs, bones or vessels): indirect signs are indications for shock (rapid pulse, low blood pressure, altered consciousness, cold sweat; see Page 41), probably visible swelling because of in-bleeding (e.g. at the thigh in case of broken bone; rarely visible at the abdominal area)

What can happen?
- Shock (see Page 41)

What to do?
Exterior bleeding: stop it before taking any other measures (e.g. resuscitation)
- Immediately apply pressure to the wound (compress, towel, hand)
- Bleeding of a limb: raise limb
- Apply pressure bandage (see fig. 5)
- Check the bandage for bleed-through (it should remain intact): check for blue skin discoloration or tingling sensation

⚠️ Constriction (tourniquet, blood pressure cuff) is not recommended because of possible tissue damage. In case of interior bleeding, it is essential to get medical attention as soon as possible—there are no options here for medical novices!

How to do – Apply Pressure Bandage
- Place bandage or wound pressure pack onto the damaged area
- Wrap gauze bandage around the wounded limb
- Place non-absorbing part (e.g. packed gauze bandage, pack of tissues) below the cloth/scarf/towel and knot tightly over the wound

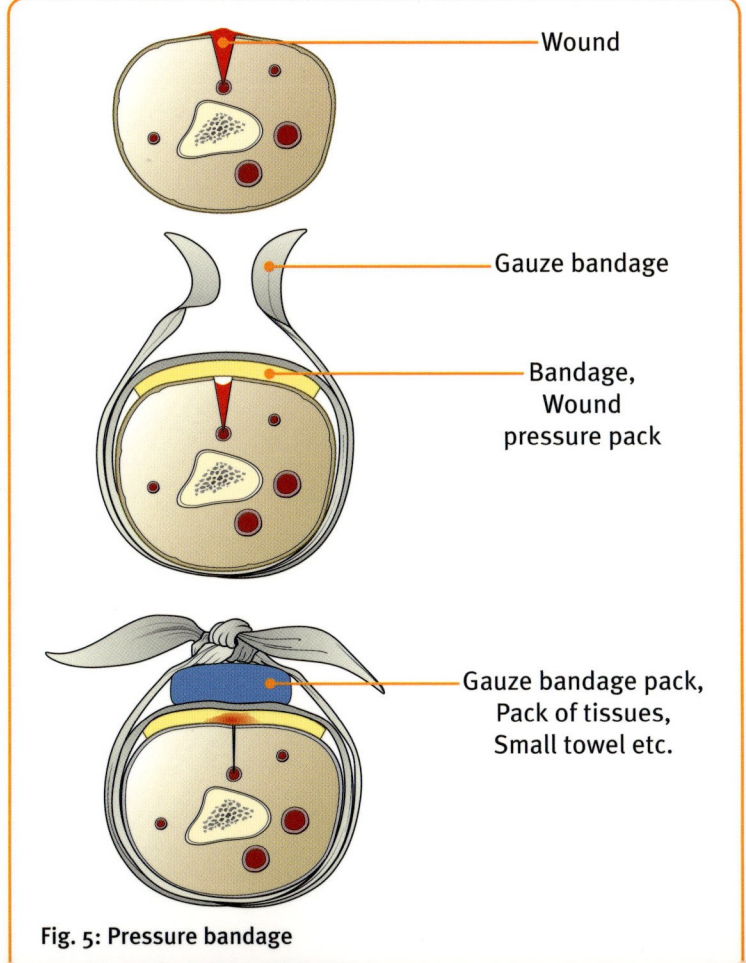

Fig. 5: Pressure bandage

Life-threatening Situations – Severe Breathing Difficulties

Causes
- Swallowing an object (e.g. food, toys in case of children)
- Inflammation of the windpipe due to insect bite or sting, or an allergic reaction
- Pneumothorax due to accident with injury of the thorax, or after scuba diving
- Other causes: See Page 36, Main Symptom–Breathing Difficulty and chest pain

How to recognize?
- **Severe breathing difficulties:** Rapid and shallow breathing, rapid pulse, increasing impaired consciousness, gray or bluish skin discoloration, panic
- **Foreign object:** Progression within seconds, foreign object might be visible, strong coughing and choking, absent breathing sound
- **Inflammation:** Progression within minutes, visible sting or bite, visible inflammation of the mouth/throat area, known allergy
- **Pneumothorax:** Rapid progression or over a period of time, after injury to the thorax or scuba diving, continually deteriorating general state of health, hollow sound when tapping the affected side (see Page 16)

What can happen?
- Panic
- Impaired consciousness, unconsciousness

What to do?
In all cases of breathing difficulties:
- Calm down patient
- Remove constricting clothing
- Observe carefully
- Check pulse and blood pressure
- Annotate examination results (protocol)
- Apply position for patients with breathing difficulty (see Page 39)

In case of breathing difficulties due to object:
- Encourage coughing
- Hit between the shoulder blades
- "Heimlich"-maneuver (see fig. 6, page 15)

Breathing difficulties due to inflammation (insect sting/bite, allergy):
- Suck on ice
- Gargle cold beverage
- Apply wet scarf

Life-threatening Situations – Severe Breathing Difficulties

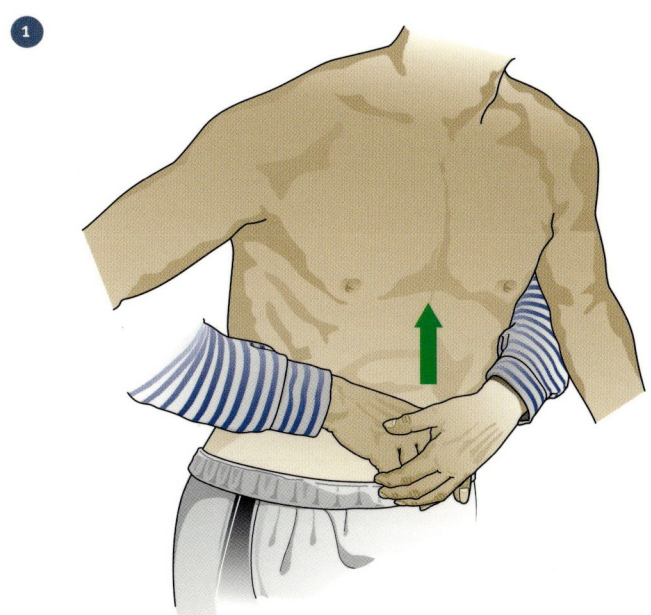
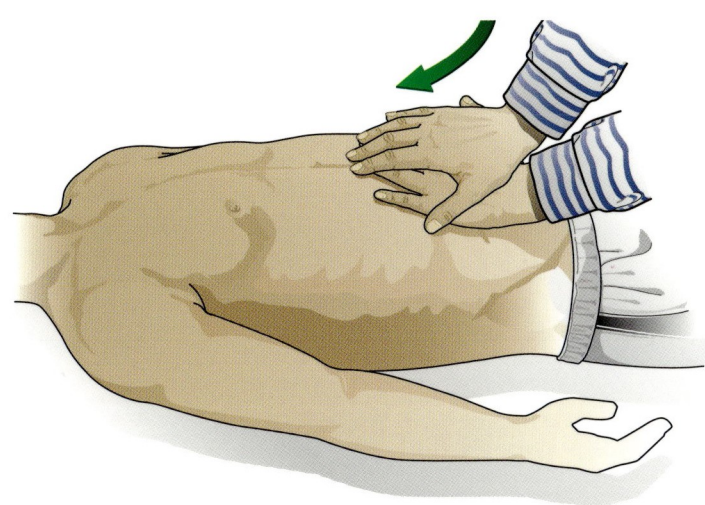

Fig. 6: The Heimlich-maneuver

① Standing upright:
- Grab patient from behind with both arms.
- Lock hands and perform a strong movement towards the inside and upwards to expel foreign object.

② Lying down:
- Place both hands onto the sternum and strongly press towards the chest.

⚠ The Heimlich maneuver causes a significant pressure increase in the upper abdomen towards the head; the intention is to expel foreign objects. However, there is a danger of damage to organs. Do not perform with children!

In case of breathing difficulties due to pneumothorax:

In the case of pneumothorax, air enters the chest after an injury or pre-existing illness from the outside or the inside and causes the collapse of the affected lung.

Simple form: Painful, usually no complications, no significant deterioration of the general state of health.
↘ Apply painkiller
↘ Physical rest

Complex form (valvular or tension pneumothorax): Increasing air volume in the chest causes increasing displacement of lung, heart, and large blood vessels (Fig. 7-1). Pronounced deterioration of general state of health; lethal if left untreated!
↘ In case of visible wound to the chest: Apply plastic film bandage (Fig. 7-2); there are no other treatment options for medical novices.

In case of breathing difficulties with unconsciousness:
↘ See Page 7 (Life-threatening Situations)

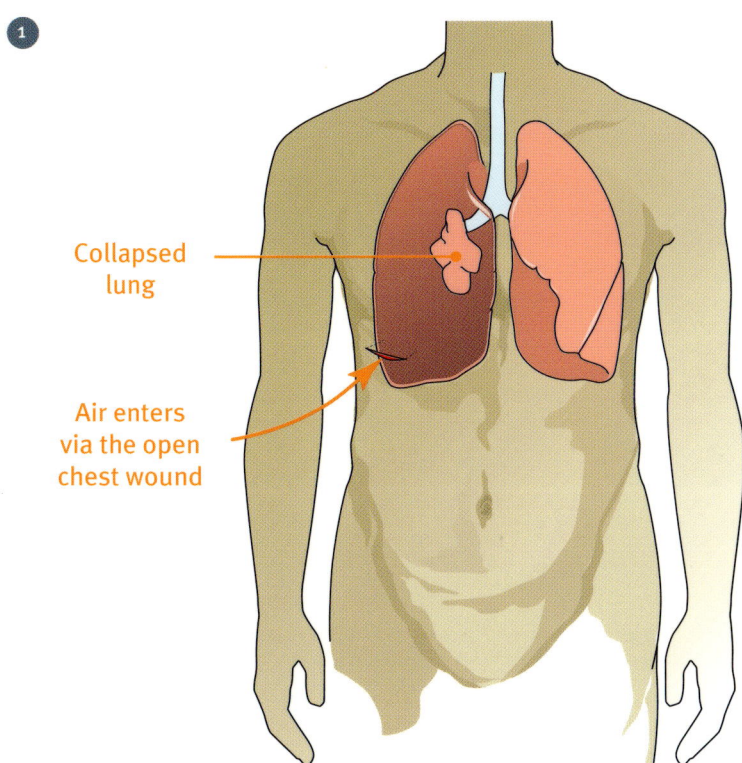

❶ Complex pneumothorax – Mechanism

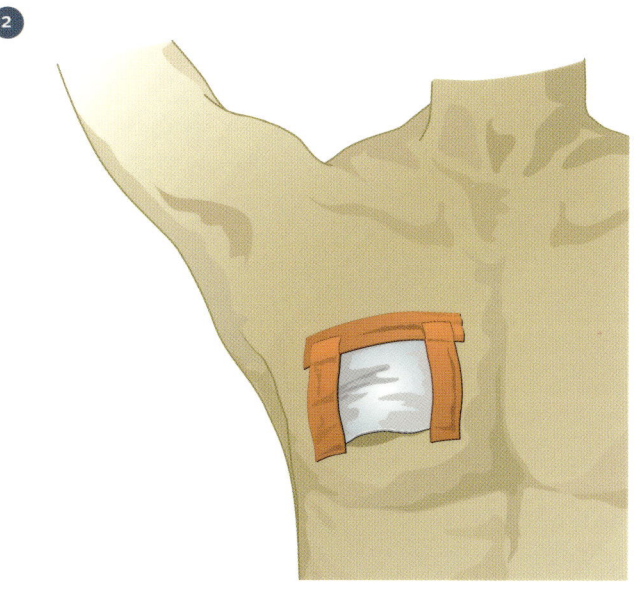

❷ Plastic film bandage: Existing (non-airtight) bandages are removed or taped over with a plastic film, affixed at three of its sides. **Effect:** Air can escape to the outside when exhaling (too much pressure inside of the chest), while when inhaling (negative pressure) the film is aspirated and minimizes the intake of air.

Fig. 7: Pneumothorax

Life-threatening Situations – Self-endangerment due to Impaired Consciousness

Causes
- Impaired circulation in the brain (e.g. stroke, bleeding)
- Psychiatric disorder (e.g. mental illness)
- Consumption or withdrawal symptoms of alcohol or other drugs
- Seizure

How to recognize?
- Impaired consciousness: reduced or increased activity
- Unimpaired consciousness but marked behavioral abnormalities
- Both can lead to self-endangerment or that of the environment

What can happen?
- Inflated self-esteem, misinterpretation, disorientation
- Absent reflexes, weakness, coordination difficulties
- Aggressiveness (towards oneself or other persons)

What to do?
- Remove person from danger zone: See Page 6 (Rescue grip)
- Prevent dangerous actions via immobilization
- Calm down patient
- Continuous observation
- Do not allow yourself to be provoked
- In case of seizure: Avoid injuries, remove objects, protect patient with pillow.

 Caution: Do not use bite blocks – risk of injury!

- In case of altered vital signs: See Page 6
- In case of hypothermia: See Page 49
- Drugs: See Page 67 and following

The Examination

The examination is the prerequisite for any treatment. The goal of the examination is the collection of information. A medical consultation may result in a diagnosis to determine the kind of treatment.

How to do
1. Annotate examination and results ("Examination" form)
2. If necessary, ask for medical consultation ("Radio-assisted Consultation" form)
3. Perform diagnosis (or have it performed)
4. Treatment
5. If necessary, repeat examination ("Protocol")

A patient may be examined with or without aid or resources. The results are compared with standard values or levels (see chart). Deviations are possible without indicating illness: Athletes, for example, have a slower pulse than untrained persons, patients with high blood pressure might not at all feel well with "normal" levels. This is why the clinical history is always important ("Medical Information" form).

Standard Values

Standard values for breathing, pulse, and blood pressure for adults and children

Age	1 year*	5 years*	12 years*	adults
Breathing frequency (per minute)	35	25	12–15	
Pulse (per minute)	110	80	70	60–80
Upper blood pressure (mm Hg)	100	100	110	110 + (Age/3)

* Values for awake children

Good to know
- Individual deviations are common!
- Each inhalation is counted to determine breathing frequency.
- Adjust blood pressure cuffs to the size of the patient (cuffs for children!), otherwise wrong data may result.
- Fever: The pulse increases by about 20 per minute for each degree (Celsius) of increased temperature.

IMPORTANT

- Examinations require training, so practice with healthy people before a journey or trip!
- Every passenger should compile information about his or her own medical history and turn it over to the captain ("Medical information" form).
- Perform some of the examinations (e.g. tapping, signs of decreased heart performance, skin creases) to compare with your own or other healthy passengers.
- Questioning and performing an examination may be stressful for the patient. Make sure you establish an undisturbed environment and ask other people to leave.
- Make detailed annotations including the time of day ("Examination" form).

Examination Methods
❶ Questions **❸** Examination without aid
❷ Observe and Listen **❹** Examination with aid

❶ Questions
- What is the problem? Where? Since when?
- Which one of the symptoms bothers you most?
- Do you feel pain?
  - When? (Always, when moving, before/after meals?)
  - Where? (Have it shown to you)
  - How? (Dull-piercing, stingy, wave-like?)
- Do you suffer from pre-existing conditions?
- Did you experience the current symptoms before? What was the treatment?
- Do you take medication (Regularly, under certain circumstances)?
- Do you suffer from allergies?
- Evacuation? Urine? (Time of day, smell and color)

> **IMPORTANT**
>
> Ask simple questions, if necessary, specific questions ("Where does it hurt?", "Since when?", "Did you have these complaints before?") or neutral questions ("And what happened then?", "What caught your attention?"). Do not ask suggestive questions ("Could this be due to the food?")

❷ Observe and Listen
Important: Do not focus on what seems to be the important issue; you should rather try to get an overall picture in order to not miss any facts.
- What is the general state of health? Normal? Reduced? Bad?
- How is the posture: Straight? Curved?
- What is the skin like? Pale or bluish? Dry or soaked with sweat? Differences in color and temperature from one side to the other?
- Signs of inflammation: reddening/blushing? Inflammation? Pains? Functionally impaired? Smell? Visible puss?

❸ Examination without Aid
Many types of examinations can be performed without any aid. Some of them are simple (dehydration, check strength and sensitivity, nail test); others require experience (checking pulse, check for signs of thrombosis, tap the chest or the stomach).

Indicators for Dehydration
Dehydration is often the result of altered or impaired consciousness, shock, or too much sun exposure.

How to do:
- Take a section of skin and lift it up, then let it go: What happens?
- Examine the tongue: Is it dry? Compare with healthy subject.
- Examine urine: Reduced amount? Dark color?
- Examine pulse and blood pressure: Rapid pulse? Low blood pressure?

Possible results:
"Standing skin fold" after release (Fig. 8), a dry tongue, small amounts of strongly colored urine and a rapid pulse are indications of dehydration.

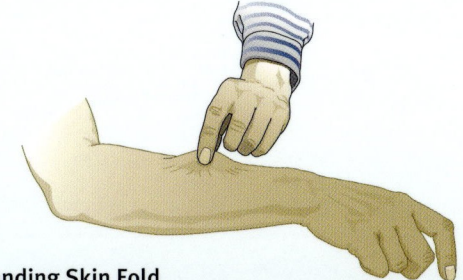

Fig. 8: Standing Skin Fold

Additional Examination without Aid
- Check sensitivity, strength, and mobility, Page 21
- Check pulse, Page 23
- Check heart function with nail test, Page 23
- Feel and tap, chest Page 24; stomach, Page 28
- Check for signs of thrombosis, Page 25
- Perform body check, Page 30

❹ Examination with Aid
Aids are either simple to use (thermometer, wooden spatula) or difficult to use (blood pressure cuff, stethoscope, quick tests). It only makes sense to bring them along if their use has been thoroughly practiced!

Measuring temperature
The body temperature is part of the basic information.

How to do:
↘ The most accurate measurements are at the rectum and the eardrum.

At least one non-battery operated and mercury-free thermometer and one automatic or manual blood pressure cuff should be on board.

Possible Results:
↘ 96-98ºF (35.5–37ºC): Normal result (lowest results in the early morning hours)
↘ 95ºF (35ºC) and less: Hypothermia
↘ From 99.5ºF (37.5ºC): High Temperature
↘ From 100.4ºF (38ºC): Fever

Additional Examination with Aid
- Note change of pupils, Page 22
- Measure changes of blood sugar, Page 22
- Examine mouth and throat, Page 25
- Measure blood pressure, Page 26
- Use stethoscope to check chest, Page 26; stomach, Page 29
- Apply troponin quick test, Page 27
- Apply urine test strips, Page 29

Examining Consciousness and Nervous System: Questions
Information regarding impaired orientation, sensitivity, and strength, as well as its localization, is important for types of impaired consciousness.

How to do – Ask for ...
↘ Name
↘ Date of birth
↘ Current location
↘ Today's date

Possible Results:
↘ Patient responds to all questions correctly: Normal result
↘ Patient answers the wrong way or not at all: Indication for impaired or altered consciousness

Examining Consciousness and Nervous System: Watch and Listen
↘ Check alertness (vigilance): Talk to – shake – check pain threshold (pinching)
↘ Other indications? Altered expression? Drooping lips? Can patient whistle?
↘ New speech impairment? Slurring, unclear speaking, nonsensical speaking, problem finding words?
↘ New visual impairment? Double images, blurred vision, blindness
↘ Dilation of pupils? Slow or no reaction of the pupils to light? (Page 22)

Examination Consciousness and Nervous System: Without Aid

Sensitivity
How to do?
- Patient closes eyes
- Examiner touches or pinches one of the patient's toes or fingers and asks: "Which toe/finger am I touching?"

Possible Results:
- Patient gives correct answer: Normal result
- Patient cannot give correct answer: Sensitivity is impaired, e.g. in the case of neurological illness (paralysis) or after a slipped/herniated disc

Stiff neck
How to do?
Move the head forward towards the sternum.

Possible results:
- The head can be moved towards the chest without pain: Normal result
- The head cannot be moved or causes pain when moved towards the chest: This is often the case when the neck muscles are contracted, stiff neck (meningismus, Fig. 9), in case of meningitis.

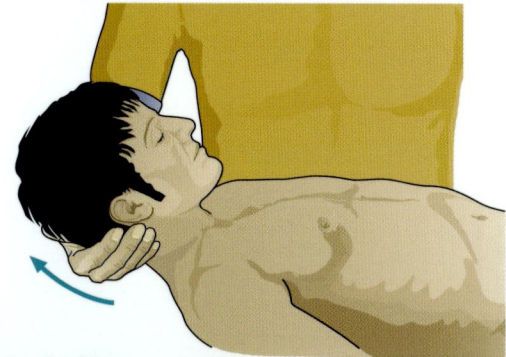

Fig. 9: Meningismus

Strength and Mobility
How to do?
Different areas of the body are checked comparing sides: handshake, lift legs, move toes against resistance towards the head (Fig. 10)

Possible Results:
- Strength is equal on both sides: Normal result
- Diminished strength on one side: In case of neurological illness (e.g. paralysis) or after a herniated disc

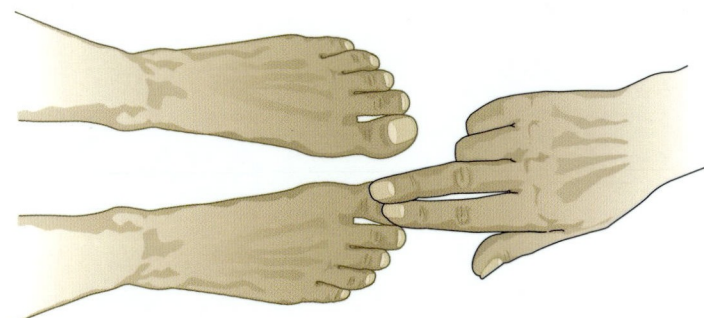

Fig. 10: Strength test

Examining Consciousness and Nervous System: With Aid

Change of Pupil
How to Do?
Indicate to close eyes or close them, open eyes and observe reaction to light (Aid: Flashlight for pupils)

Possible Results:
- Pupils are the same size: Normal result
- Pupils are a different size: Indicates impaired consciousness (Page 33) or possibly grave cerebral damage (Fig. 11)

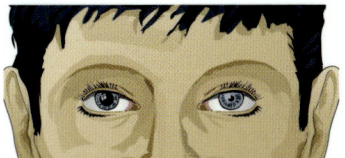

Fig. 11: Different Pupils

 **TIP** — **Aid: Pupil Flashlight:** Used to determine the size of the pupils or to examine the throat (Page 25). Any flashlight is suitable as long as it is not too bright.

Changes in Blood Sugar
Changes in the blood sugar can cause impaired consciousness. Usually the blood sugar testing device is suitable for regular controls in case of blood sugar illness; it is supposed to exclude excessive or too little blood sugar as the cause of impaired consciousness.

Measuring Blood Sugar – How to Do?
- Remove a drop of blood: Pinch the tip of a finger with a hypodermic needle, pull back syringe.
- Hold test strip to the drop of blood.
- Follow the instructions on the device

Possible Results:
- 75–150 mg%: normal result
- below 70 mg%: low blood sugar
- over 250 mg%: blood sugar too high (consultation!)

Important:
The test must be practiced! Important variations are possible with respect to the effects of too much or too little blood sugar. Diabetics must show fellow passengers how to perform blood sugar measurements.

Examining Breathing Passages, Respiration, Heart and Blood Circulation: Questions
- **Breathing Passages:** Obstructed nose? Sensation of insufficient air when breathing?
- **Chest Pain:** Getting stronger when coughing or breathing deeply? Does the pain project into the left arm, shoulder, back, or neck? Panic? Fear of death? Sensation of constricted chest? Nausea?
- **Existing Risk of Thrombosis?** (Impaired mobility when resting in bed? Injury with swelling? Irregular heartbeat?)

Examining Breathing Passages, Respiration, Heart and Blood Circulation: Listen and Observe
- **Skin:** Sweating? **Face and Lips:** Red or pale?
- **Breathing Passages:** Coughing? With or without mucus? What color is the mucus?
- **Breathing:** Regular? Deeper? Difficulty? No audible breathing (Page 24)?
- **Breathing Frequency:** Too low or too high (counting the inhalations)?
- **Chest:** Visible injury? Hematoma?

Examining Breathing Passages, Respiration, Heart, and Blood Circulation: Without Aid

Feeling the Pulse
Information regarding pulse is part of the basic information.

How to do?
- Place index and middle finger (not the thumb!) and press lightly onto the thumb-side of the lower arm (Fig. 12a), the groin, the neck, or next to the Achilles tendon at the inside of the ankle (Fig. 12b)
- Count the pulse per minute

Possible Result:
- Pulse even (60-80/min): Normal result
- Pulse uneven: Cardiac arrhythmia
- Pulse slow (<---60/min): Cardiac arrhythmia, normal with athletes
- Pulse rapid (--->100/min): Shock, normal after physical exercise
- No pulse: Circulatory arrest, low blood pressure, wrong examination technique

> **IMPORTANT**
>
> Feeling the pulse takes practice — in case of emergency, do not waste time! See chart on Page 18 for normal pulse values.

Check Heart Strength
Information regarding heart strength is part of the basic medical information.

Indications for diminished heart strength:
- Nail test takes longer
- Blood vessels at the neck are swollen and more visible than usual
- Ankles are swollen on both sides
- Moist-burbling breathing sound can be heard, probably with coughing and white-foamy mucus (indicates pulmonary edema)
- Rapid pulse, low blood pressure

How to Do – Nail Test
- Place the patient's fingernail onto a hard surface (e.g. a desk).
- Press fingernail strongly onto the surface (Fig. 13) so that the tissue under the fingernail turns whitish
- Release and observe red coloration.

Possible Results:
- Quick red coloration (ca. 2 seconds) after release: Normal result
- Extended time until red color returns: Diminished heart strength

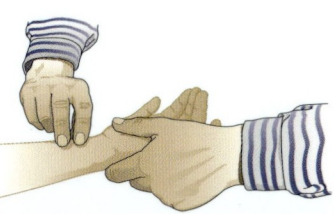

Fig. 12a: Checking pulse at the wrist

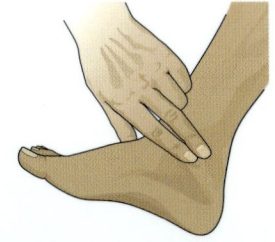

Fig. 12b: Checking pulse at the ankle

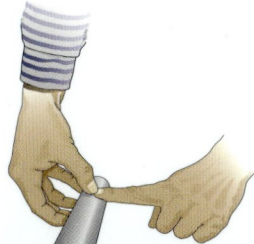

Fig. 13: Nail Test

⚠ The nail test is not reliable in case of hypothermia! Always compare with a healthy person.

Checking the Chest

How to do?
- Place hands with fingers flat just below the collarbone – best with a reclining patient (Fig. 14).
- Check: Existing breathing? Breathing frequency (number of inhalations)? Are both sides of the lung active? Is the chest moving on both sides while breathing? Is the breathing uneven, meaning the chest does not move to the outside on one side but rather, it is pulled inwards? Is the blood pressure unstable? Does the skin crinkle when applying pressure?

Possible Results:
- Normal result: See chart on Page 18
- No noticeable movement: Very shallow breathing or no breathing
- One side does not move: Pneumonia, pneumothorax, obstruction of one lung due to foreign object
- The skin "crinkles" or "sizzles" with stronger pressure (check at several locations): Pneumothorax
- The chest is unstable, probable crinkling or sizzling: Broken rib, perhaps with open wound
- Paradoxical breathing: Broken rib

Tapping the Chest

How to do?
- Place the fingers of the hand to be tapped flat onto the chest of the sitting or reclining patient (Fig. 15).
- Use a quick and swift movement from the wrist with one or two fingers of the other hand and tap onto the middle finger of the flat hand. The audible sound depends on the air and fluid content inside the chest and the lung.
- Check: Is one half of the lung impaired in its function due to air or fluid (inside the chest, outside of the lung)?

Possible Results:
- Tapping sound "normal," just like tapping a piece of wood on a hard surface: Normal result, both sides of the lung are filled with air.
- Hollow sound, like tapping an empty bottle: There is an increased amount of air on this side of the chest, e.g. in case of a pneumothorax.
- Sound is dampened, such as tapping a large muscle: There is a diminished amount of air on this side of the chest, the content of fluid may be increased such as in case of pneumonia or bleeding inside the chest.

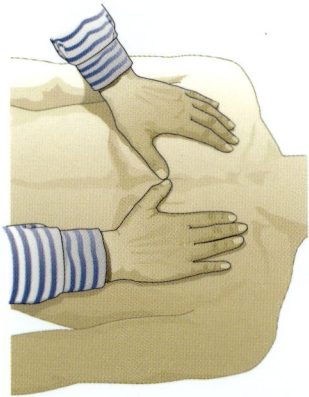

Fig. 14: Checking and feeling the chest: Examining chest movement

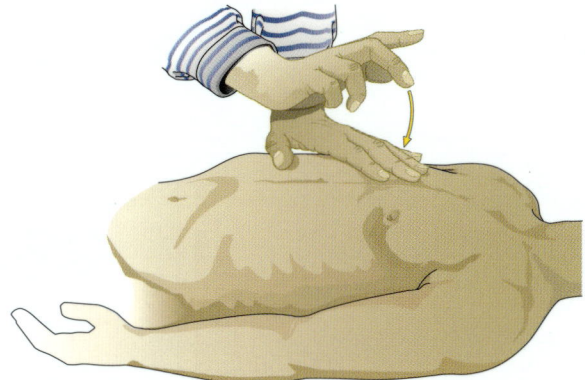

Fig. 15: Tapping the Chest

Check Signs for Thrombosis

How to do?
- Compare calves: Is one of them swollen and painful?
- Does the pain increase when massaging the calf, bending the foot towards the head or when applying a blow with the edge of the palm onto the base of the foot (Fig. 16)?

Possible Results:
- No pain, no swelling: Normal result
- Swelling, pain during the examination: Vein obstruction (thrombosis)

> **IMPORTANT**
>
> Always follow up on signs of a vein obstruction. Should the blood clot dissolve and be carried into the lung, then a life-threatening pulmonary embolism can result (Page 40).

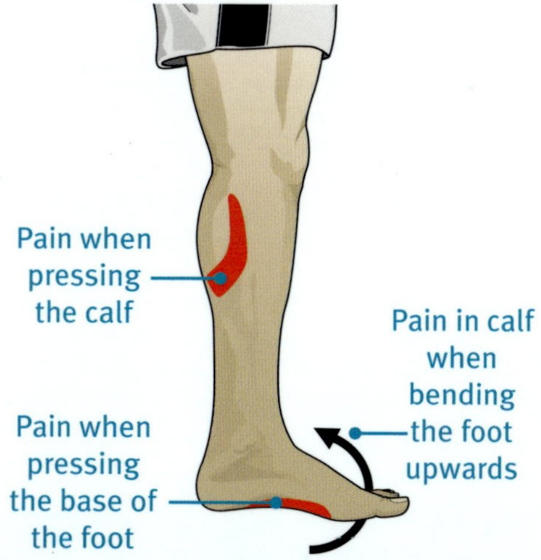

Examination of Mouth and Throat

Colds are rather common on board and usually caused by viruses. Illnesses caused by bacteria must be treated with antibiotics.

How to do?
- In Case of Tonsillitis: Stipples in the throat area (Fig. 17)
  - Have patient open mouth and say "Aaaa ... "
  - Use flashlight and wooden spatula to examine the rear throat area
- In Case of Sinusitis: Pain when tapping over the sinuses and frontal sinuses
  - Use a quick movement from the wrist to tap different points (Fig. 18)
- In Case of Infection of the Middle Ear: Pains and cracking sounds when swallowing
- Additionally: Yellow mucus, high fever for more than 3 days

Possible Results:
- No stipples, no pain when tapping, no mucus, no fever: Normal result or common cold
- Stipples, tapping pain, fever, mucus, "cracking" sound when swallowing: Bacterial inflammation of the breathing passages

Fig. 16: Signs of thrombosis: Pain areas in case of vein obstruction.

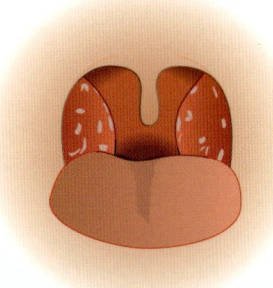

Fig. 17: Stipples inside the throat in case of bacterial tonsillitis

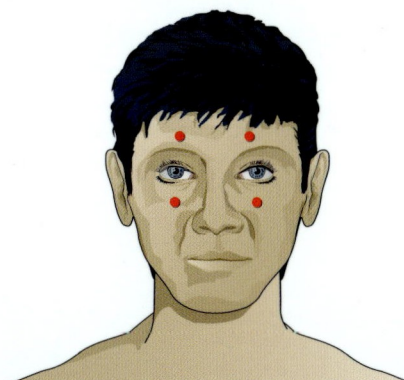

Fig. 18: Tapping points for Sinusitis

Measuring Blood Pressure

Taking blood pressure measurements is part of the basic information. The measurement of the upper (systolic) blood pressure is sufficient. The measurement does not need a stethoscope and is performed by feeling the pulse.

How to do?
- Put cuff around upper arm.
- Inflate cuff while continually feeling the pulse until no pulse is audible anymore. Feel pulse at the lower arm (Fig. 19).
- Slowly (!) decrease pressure. The value when you feel the pulse again corresponds to the upper value.

Possible Results:
- Normal findings: See table on page 18.
- Low blood pressure: Heart attack, heart weakness, or shock. **Important:** A low blood pressure is only detrimental if other problems are present (e.g. nausea, fainting, fatigue).
- Heightened blood pressure: As a chronic illness in case of high blood pressure crisis. **Important:** With existing high blood pressure levels, higher levels can be "normal," e.g. an upper value of 160 mm Hg.

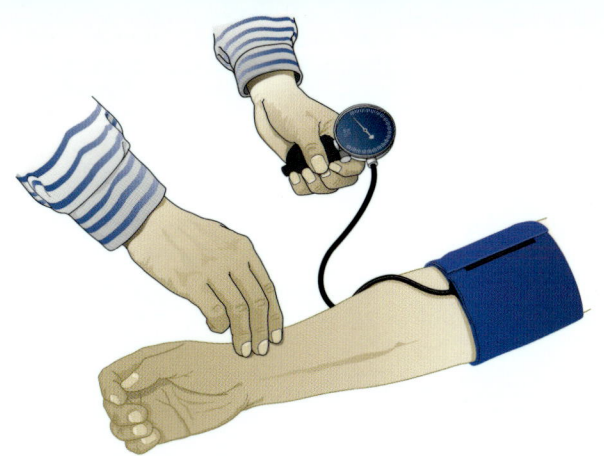

Fig. 19: Manual blood pressure measurement

IMPORTANT

The manual measurement can always be performed and it is independent of batteries. Alternatively, a manual blood pressure cuff should always be on board. Use as indicated. The results are not as exact (particularly in case of low blood pressures), however, they are easier to use.

Examining the Chest with a Stethoscope

How to do?
- Press the membrane of the stethoscope firmly next to the nipples and listen for breathing sound (Fig. 20).

Possible Results:
- Audible breathing sounds at both sides: Normal result
- No audible breathing sounds on one side: The affected side is not receiving air (e.g. in case of acute breathing difficulty, Page 14)
- No audible breathing sounds on both sides: Shallow or no breathing

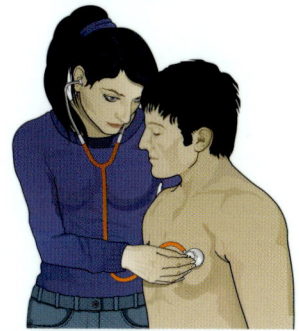

Fig. 20: Checking the chest with a stethoscope

IMPORTANT

It is difficult to handle a stethoscope accurately, so be careful when assessing the results!

Using the Troponin Quick Test
How to do?
- Draw blood from a vein: Constrict blood flow at one arm (with blood pressure cuff or rubber hose); use a hollow needle to draw blood into a small (2 ml) syringe.
- Follow the instructions of the test (Fig. 21).

Possible Results:
The test can discard or confirm a heart attack.

IMPORTANT

This procedure must be practiced beforehand!

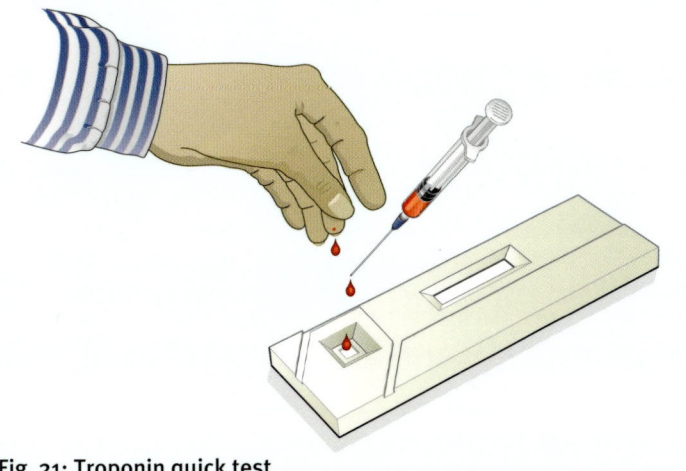

Fig. 21: Troponin quick test

Examination of the Abdomen: Questions
- Where does it hurt? When did it begin hurting? Describe the pain (permanent, wave-like, light or dark pain)?
- Burning pain when urinating?
- Existing appetite?
- Nausea after ingesting coffee, fat foods, chocolate, alcohol?
- Noticeable stool: Color, consistency, bloody?
- Diarrhea: How often?
- Vomit: Color, bloody, stool-like smell?
- Simultaneous vomiting and diarrhea?
- Do other passengers have similar problems?

Examining the Stomach: Listen and Watch
- Relieving Posture (Fig. 22): Bent upper body, bent legs?
- Stomach with spherical swelling?
- Yellow discoloration of the eyes?
- Protrusions in the groin area, at the navel, at the testicles? Indications for hernias (e.g. umbilical hernia)
- Intestinal noises (place your ear on the body and listen for one minute)? Gurgling noises several times a minute, increased frequency in the case of diarrhea, and at the start of an intestinal obstruction, no noise in case of (generalized) inflammations affecting the entire body (e.g. peritonitis)

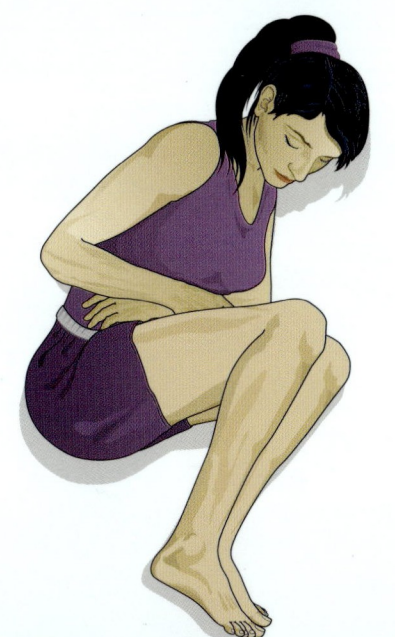

Fig. 22: Relieving Posture

Examining the Stomach: Without Aid
Looking for signs of a possibly serious illness.

Feeling the Stomach
How to do?
- Place the hands with the fingers flat just below the ribs; press the fingertips into the abdomen with increasing pressure.
  Note: If general changes are not noticeable, localize within a quadrant (Fig. 23).
- A blow with the side of the hand: Use the edge of the hand hitting both sides of the flank (Fig. 24).

Possible Results:
- Abdomen is soft, free of pain, and not swollen: Normal result
- Abdomen is sensitive to the touch with increasing pressure: Inflammation
- Abdomen with spherical inflammation: Intestinal obstruction, increased gas formation
- Abdomen is "as hard as a board" (Fig. 24): Peritonitis
- Pain when applying side of hand blow (Fig. 24): Indicates kidney disease (Page 46)
- Typical pain at the points of pain (Fig. 24) in case of gall bladder disorders and urinary retention

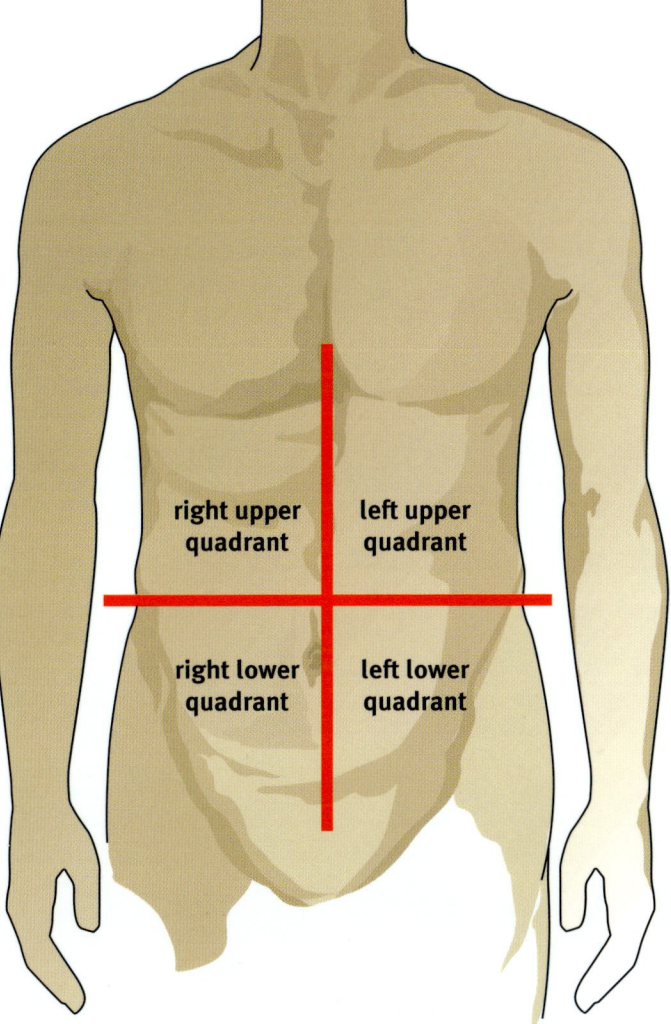

Fig. 23: Division of the abdomen into quadrants

Indications for Appendicitis

How to do?
1. Use one finger to press deeply into the area with pain (Fig. 24, between 1 and 2)
2. The reclining patient raises his leg against resistance

Possible Results:
1. Pain at the pain location
2. Abdominal pain when contracting muscles.

> **IMPORTANT**
>
> Appendicitis is common and dangerous!

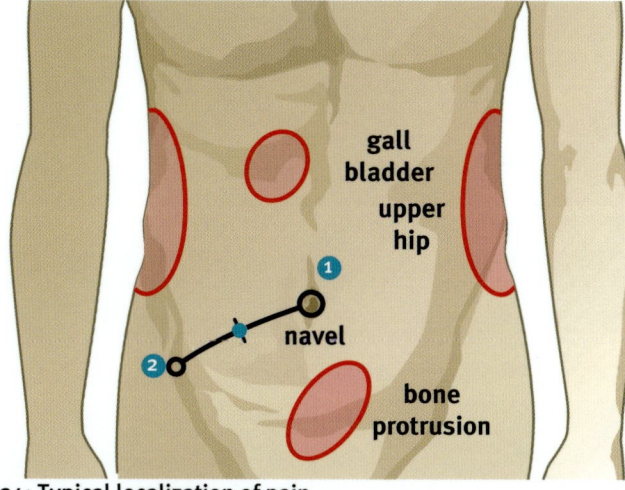

Fig. 24: Typical localization of pain.

Examining the Abdomen: With Aid

Examining the Abdomen with Stethoscope

How to do?
- Place the membrane of the stethoscope firmly onto the skin just below the navel and listen for about one minute.
- Check: Are there existing intestinal noises?

Possible Results:
- See Page 27

> **IMPORTANT**
>
> Handling a stethoscope is difficult—practice before the voyage!

Using Urine Test Strips

How to do?
- Collect urine
- Insert test strip
- Determine change of color
- Check: Could an inflammation of the bladder be a possible cause for flank or abdominal pain, or burning pain when urinating?

Possible Results:
- See color markings on the package

 TIP The test with urine strips makes it possible to decide for or against the use of antibiotics.

Body-Check After an Accident

In the case of unclear accident details, or when there is a possibility of major injuries, then a full body-check should be performed. The goal is to not miss a potentially dangerous injury.

> **IMPORTANT**
>
> In all cases of injuries to the locomotor system: Start icing the area as soon as possible!

Important Basic Information

How did the injury occur? Is it due to an accident, such as getting hit by a falling beam, due to an illness, or injury such as a fall after suddenly fainting? An illness can be much more of a serious problem than a possible injury due to the accident or fall. Examine as described above after checking the following questions (see also Pages 31 and 54).

Are immediate measures necessary?
- Are vital parameters affected? See Page 6 and following
- Profuse bleeding? Apply pressure bandage if necessary (Page 13)
- Fall with possible head or neck/spine injury? Apply immobilizing collar (Page 59)

Questions
- What happened? Can you remember everything?
- Where does it hurt?
- Can you move your entire body? Please move … (indicate to slowly move all extremities)
- Check orientation: Ask for name, birth date, current location, and today's date.

How to do? – Body-Check
- The examination is performed from the head to the feet using your hands.
- Examine first without causing pain: Start by using little strength and increase strength if there is no pain.
- In case of indications for an injury, remove restrictive clothing.

Possible Results

Examination from head to feet:
- **Head:** Wounds, pupils, swelling? Hold head with both hands and press.
- **Neck:** Noticeable swelling in the area of the neck vertebrae?
- **Chest:** Press sternum from both sides, paradoxical breathing (Page 24)?
- **Arms and hands:** Deformation, swelling, compression pain? Press the extended arm from the hand towards the shoulder.
- **Abdomen:** Soft? Visible injuries, swelling?
- **Hip:** Apply pressure on the pubic bone and, with both hands, on the pelvis shovels.
- **Legs and feet:** Deformations, swelling, compression pain? Press the extended leg from the foot towards the hip. Difference in length of leg?

Indicators for Shock (Page 41):
- Low blood pressure
- Fast pulse
- Paleness
- Lowered heart strength

Examination of the Injured Area:
- Check blood flow: Feel pulse after the injury and perform nail test (Page 23). Is the area after the injury cool and pale? Is there nerve damage or functional impairment due to swelling?
- Check sensitivity after the injury (Page 21): Damaged blood vessel or impaired functionality due to swelling?
- Check for compartment syndrome (Page 56): Swelling? Impaired sensitivity?

Guiding Symptoms and Illnesses

Guiding Symptoms

Illness and disease lead to problems and signs (symptoms). Prominent symptoms are called guiding symptoms:
- Impaired consciousness
- Breathing difficulty
- Chest pain
- Abdominal pain

Examine the patient as described in the previous chapter. A systematic examination can result in a diagnosis. Annotate your results in the forms "Examination" and "Protocol" (Page 82). Typical findings are given; however, they may be absent. Instructions regarding treatment with medication can be found starting on Page 67. In case your travel first-aid kit varies, make sure you apply your own labeling.

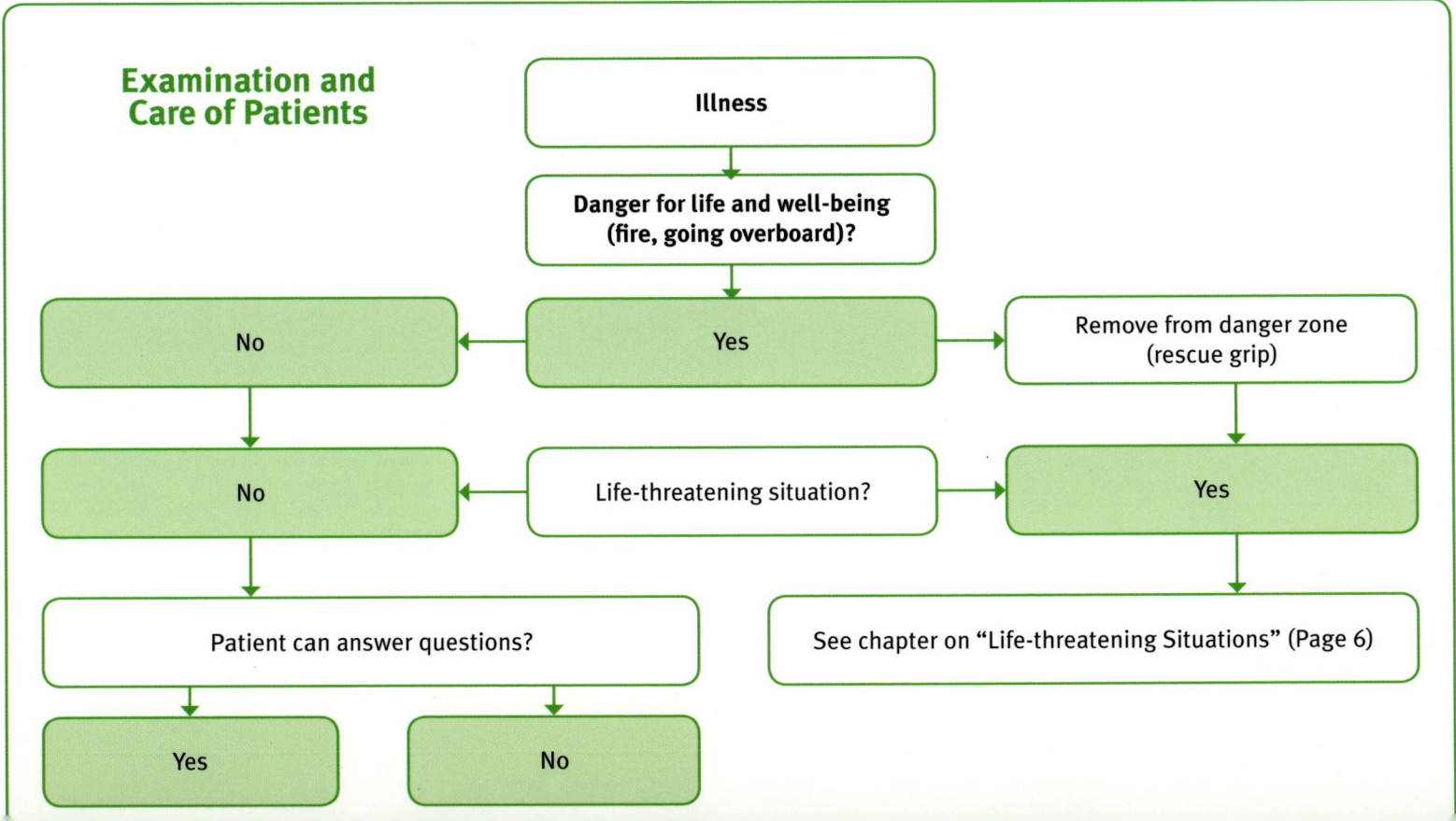

Examination and Care of Patients

Illness → Danger for life and well-being (fire, going overboard)?
- No → Life-threatening situation?
  - No → Patient can answer questions? → Yes / No
- Yes → Remove from danger zone (rescue grip) → Life-threatening situation?
  - Yes → See chapter on "Life-threatening Situations" (Page 6)

Collect information:
- ↘ Ask for medical history
- ↘ Ask for description of main problem

Collect information:
- ↘ Ask fellow passengers
- ↘ Check health chart
- ↘ Search for medication

Initial Examination (see chapter starting on Page 18) Annotate results ("Examination" form)

Guiding Symptoms	See Page	Guiding Symptoms	See Page
Change in Consciousness	• Starting on Page 19: General examination – Consciousness and nervous system • Starting on Page 33: Guiding symptoms – impaired consciousness	**Chest Pain**	• Pages 19, 22: General examination – Respiration, heart, and circulation • Starting on Page 36: Guiding symptom – breathing difficulties and chest pain
Breathing Difficulties	• Pages 19, 22: General examination – Respiration, heart, and circulation • Starting on Page 36: Guiding symptoms – breathing difficulties and chest pain	**Abdominal Pain**	• Pages 19, 27: General examination – Abdomen • Page 44: Guiding symptom – abdominal pain
Other	• Page 19: General examination, e.g. body posture, pain, skin changes		

First Evaluation:
- ↘ Not at all – a little – very ill?
- ↘ Is immediate professional help required?
- ↘ Patient's condition: Stable – worsening condition likely?

Organize Assistance if necessary (Emergency Call, Page 5)

Determine Following Steps:
- ↘ Aid on board possible?
- ↘ Professional help on board required?
- ↘ Course change?
- ↘ Evacuation

Guiding Symptom – Impaired Consciousness

All kinds of impaired consciousness require special attention. Even after an apparent phase of improvement, a worsening situation is always possible. Persons with impaired consciousness should not be left by themselves; regular controls are important. Help with equipment on board is almost impossible. The goals are:
- Describe symptoms correctly
- Avoid situations where the condition might deteriorate
- Provide first-aid rescue if necessary (starting on Page 6)

 TIP Impaired consciousness is common in case of metabolism or neurological problems, after accidents involving the head, in case of excessive alcohol consumption, dehydration, or shock. They are also common in case of hypothermia (Page 49), sun poisoning or heat strokes (Page 50), sea-sickness (Page 74), or diseases with impaired heart strength (Page 40).

Warning Signs
- Every increasing consciousness problem
- Paralysis
- Speech impairment
- Sensitivity impairment after accident – increasing and without tendency to improve
- Impaired orientation
- Very strong headaches
- Impaired consciousness after excessive alcohol consumption – impaired respiration
- Pupils of different size
- Deep unconsciousness in case of diabetics
- New incontinence (stool and/or urine)
- Strikingly high or low blood pressure
- Impaired consciousness with stiff neck
- Seizure without prior history
- Slow breathing or pauses in breathing

What to do?
- Immediately request medical assistance!

Await First Aid
- Brief impaired consciousness after an accident
- Impaired consciousness in case of psychological commotion
- Impaired consciousness after a seizure in case of known history of seizures
- Strong headache – as previously experienced
- Impaired consciousness after excessive alcohol consumption – breathing not affected
- Slightly impaired consciousness in case of diabetics

What to do?
- Continue observation
- Treat with available equipment and/or medication

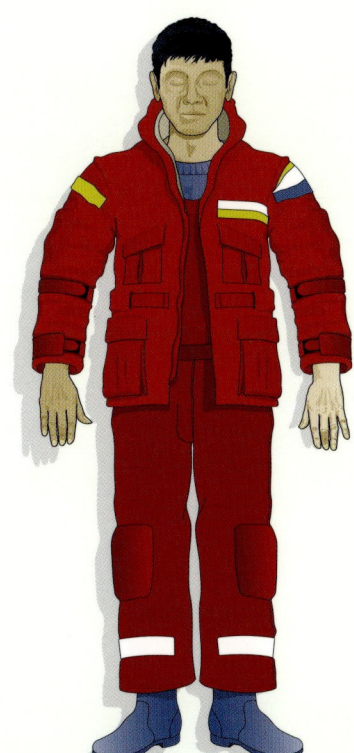

Fig. 25: Guiding Symptom – Impaired Consciousness

Illnesses and Diseases with Impaired Consciousness

Impaired Consciousness in case of Diseases or after Accidents

Causes
- Metabolism diseases: e.g. Hypothyroidism, diabetes with low blood sugar level
- Neurological diseases: Stroke, cerebral hemorrhage without an accident, meningitis, seizure (e.g. epilepsy)
- Psychiatric diseases
- Diseases with reduced heart strength (Page 40)
- Children: Fever convulsion
- Accidents: Concussion, brain hemorrhage

How to recognize?
- **Always a possibility:** Deep unconsciousness; further noticeable facts when examining consciousness and nervous system
- **In case of stroke:** Sudden onset without an accident; no headaches
- **In case of brain hemorrhage:** Probably very strong headaches "as never before"; symptoms develop immediately or over several days

TIP In case of metabolism diseases, seizures, cerebral concussion, and children's fever convulsions, there is commonly only an impairment of alertness (vigilance) without further noticeable symptoms.

- **In case of brain hemorrhage and meningitis:** Neck stiffness (Page 21, Fig. 9)
- **In case of seizure:** Illness is usually known; typical impaired consciousness and fatigue after attack
- **In case of psychiatric illness:** Noticeable behavior, e.g. delusional, aggressive, uncooperative, slow
- **In case of illness with reduced heart strength:** Indicators for reduced heart strength (Pages 23 and 40)
- **In case of metabolism diseases:** Usually known beforehand
- **In case of accidents:** Wound or hematoma at the head; symptoms range from headaches to immediate unconsciousness

What can happen?
- Unnoticed breathing arrest or circulatory arrest
- Brain damage
- Psychiatric illness: Self-endangerment
- Renewed worsening after intermittent stabilization (life-threatening!)

What to do?
- Observe, examine repeatedly, document ("Protocol" form)
- In case of doubt, always assume a serious cause
- In case of existing warning signs (Page 33): Make emergency call, get medical consultation (Page 5)
- In case of seizure: Protect patient from injuries (remove sharp objects, provide cushions)
- In case of deep unconsciousness: stable lateral position, artificial respiration, or resuscitation (Page 7)
- Unconsciousness in case of known diabetes: If possible, always provide sugar (sweet beverages, grape sugar), but never insulin without blood sugar measurement!

IMPORTANT
If psychiatric or neurological diseases are not treated optimally, they constitute one of the few pre-existing medical conditions that preclude the practice of water sports.

Impaired Consciousness due to Alcohol or Dehydration

Causes
- Excessive alcohol consumption
- Dehydration due to vomiting, diarrhea, sun poisoning, abdominal illnesses, shock, high fever

How to recognize?
- Alcohol intoxication: Consumption, smell
- Dehydration: Page 19

What can happen?
- In case of alcohol intoxication or dehydration: Deep unconsciousness
- In case of dehydration: Shock, circulatory collapse (life-threatening!)

What to do?
- In case of alcohol intoxication with remaining consciousness: Provide sweet beverages in small amounts
- In case of dehydration: Provide any type of liquid (small amounts at a time), as well as salty food
- In case of threat to life: Page 7

IMPORTANT
Do not rush to the conclusion that alcohol must be the cause for impaired consciousness; rather, first eliminate all other possibilities.

Guiding Symptoms – Breathing Difficulties and Chest Pain

TAKE NOTE

Breathing difficulties and chest pain are guiding symptoms for diseases of the lung, breathing passages, heart, and metabolism. They occur often, but are not always concurrent.

- **Breathing difficulty:** Breathing is felt to be difficult or bothersome.
- **Chest pain:** Usually the pain is localized behind the sternum.
- **Life-threatening breathing difficulties and chest pain:** In case of pneumothorax, allergic reaction (Page 14), and obstruction of the breathing passages due to a foreign object

Common Causes:
- Disease affecting lungs and breathing passages: Cold, inflammation of the lungs, worsening of an existing lung disease (asthma, bronchitis), accident with concussion of the ribs
- Heart diseases: blood pressure crisis

Rare Causes:
- Diseases of the lung and breathing passages: Pneumonia, accident with broken rib
- Diseases with reduced heart strength: Coronary syndrome, heart attack, heart weakness, cardiac arrhythmias
- Circulatory disorder: Shock, blood vessel obstruction

Warning Signs
- Breathing frequency ⇢ 30/min
- Pulse ⇠ 100/min
- Noticeably higher blood pressure
- Chest pain with concurrent nausea
- Paleness
- Sensation of chest constriction
- Panic and fear of death
- Visible injury to the chest
- Started after scuba diving
- Indications for thrombosis
- Low blood pressure
- Chest pain, radiating to other areas
- Sweating without fever
- Impaired Consciousness
- High fever
- Hard or swollen abdomen
- Known heart disease
- Known lung disease
- Worsening situation

What to do?
- Get medical assistance or consultation!

Await First Aid
- Concurrent cold
- No nausea, no sweating
- Light fever
- Good overall condition
- Normal blood pressure
- No radiating pain
- Increased pain when pressing chest
- Increased pain when breathing deeply
- Increased pain when coughing
- Known infection of the stomach (gastritis)

What to do?
- Continue observation
- Treat with medication and aid available on board

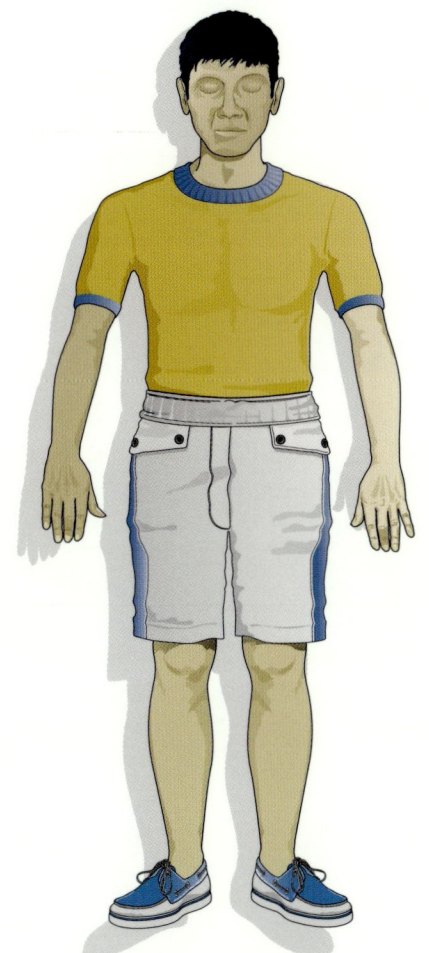

Fig. 26: Guiding symptoms – Breathing difficulties and chest pain

Illnesses and Diseases of the Lung, Breathing Passages, Heart, and Circulation

Cold and Inflammation of the Lungs (Pleurisy)

Causes
- Cold: Usually viruses and contributing wet and cold weather or unsuitable clothing. Rarely flu, Pfeiffer's disease (Mono), tonsillitis, childhood illnesses (whooping cough, measles, scarlet fever)
- Inflammation of the lungs: Complication in case of enduring cold

How to recognize?
- Headaches and neck aches
- Cough (whitish mucus), runny nose
- Limb pain, fatigue
- Fever (1–3 days)
- Irritated conjunctiva (chemosis)
- Inflammation: Pain when inhaling deeply, when coughing, and when pressing finger onto ribs

What can happen?
- Bacterial infection
- Pneumonia
- Meningitis (Page 34)
- Tonsillitis with pus (see Fig. 17)

What to do?
- In general: Rest, drink a lot of fluids
- In case of infection of the middle ear: Chew gum
- In case of inflammation: Take painkiller (inhaling and coughing should be possible without causing pain)

TIP Colds should be treated right away or complications, such as a painful middle ear infections, nasal sinuses, or inflammation, may occur. Only apply antibiotics when you have indications that a bacterial infection is present (Page 25).

Pneumonia
Causes: Infection Weak heart

How to recognize?
- Breathing difficulties are primary
- Chest pains are rather rare
- High fever Cough with yellow-green mucus
- Cold symptoms

What can happen?
- Inflammation of the lungs
- Life-threatening (!) breathing difficulties
- Dehydration due to high fever (Page 35)

What to do?
- Rest, drink a lot of fluids
- In case of increasing breathing difficulties: Position to stabilize breathing (Fig. 27)

IMPORTANT
Pneumonia is a life-threatening illness—do not underestimate!

Asthma and Bronchitis

Causes
- Chronic disease with constriction of the breathing passages
- Worsening condition often due to infection (bronchitis) or allergy (asthma)

What else could it be?
- Blood pressure crisis: Very high blood pressure
- Disease with decreased heart strength (Page 40): Signs of decreased heart strength (Page 23)
- Heart attack: Often strong pain
- Pneumonia: High fever
- Pneumothorax: Inhaling is difficult, decreased chest movement at one side

How to recognize?
- Primary problem is breathing difficulty
- Chest pains (though rather rare)
- Strong cough
- Prolonged exhalation
- "Whistling" sounds

What can happen?
- Exhaustion of the breathing muscles with increasing breathing difficulties (life-threatening!)
- Impaired consciousness up to unconsciousness

What to do?
- Calm down
- Position to stabilize (Fig. 27)

> **TAKE NOTE**
>
> If no asthma attack has occurred previously, such an attack is unlikely. Asthma or bronchitis can become life-threatening if left untreated. A radio-assisted consultation is absolutely required! If a chronic breathing passage disease is known, the location of the medication should be explained to the passengers ahead of time.

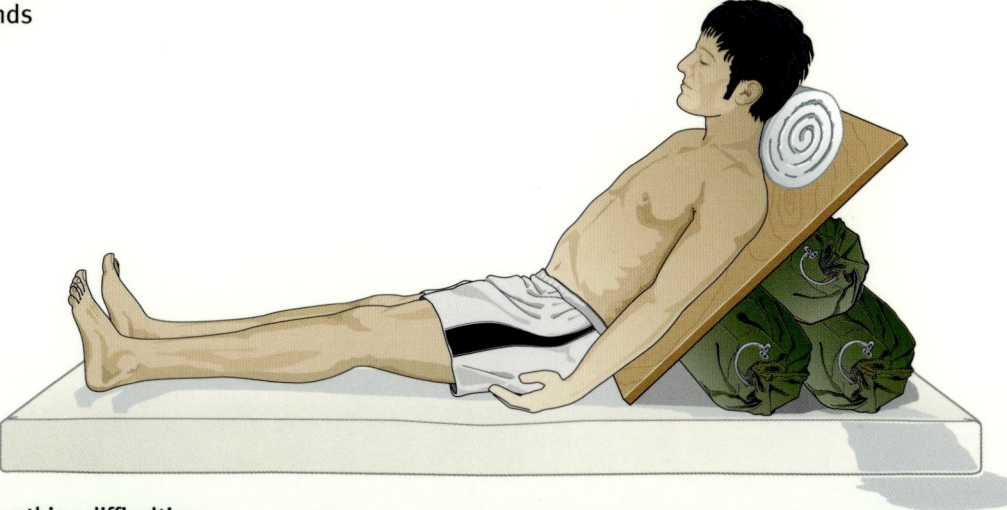

Fig. 27: Position for breathing difficulties

Diseases with Decreased Heart Strength

Causes
- Coronary syndrome (angina pectoris) with constricted coronary vessels
- Heart attack in case of obstructed coronary vessels
- Weakness of heart as a consequence of heart attack, heart asthma, pulmonary embolism, or shock
- Heart arrhythmia, either pre-existing or new, as a consequence of heart attack or pulmonary embolism

What else could it be?
- Chest pain after rib concussion, in case of muscular contraction or inflammation: The pain increases when inhaling deeply or while coughing
- Gastritis: The pain does not radiate to other areas
- Pneumothorax (Page 16)

How to recognize?
- Breathing difficulties
- Probably extreme chest pain with radiation into neck and left arm
- Panic, fear of death
- Acute coronary syndrome: Pain and other symptoms less noticeable
- Heart weakness: Pain is rare, possibly raised blood pressure
- Pulmonary embolism: Additionally, probable signs of thrombosis (Page 25)
- Cardiac arrhythmia: Feel pulse
- Other signs for decreased heart strength: Page 23

What can happen?
- Heart failure
- Shock
- Circulatory collapse (life-threatening!)
- Cardiac arrhythmia (life-threatening!)

What to do?
- Heart or breathing difficulty emergency position (Figures 27 and 28)
- Calm down
- Patient must rest
- Be prepared for resuscitation
- If available: Keep defibrillator ready

IMPORTANT
Pain may also be absent, particularly in the case of women and diabetics. Never inject medication into a muscle!

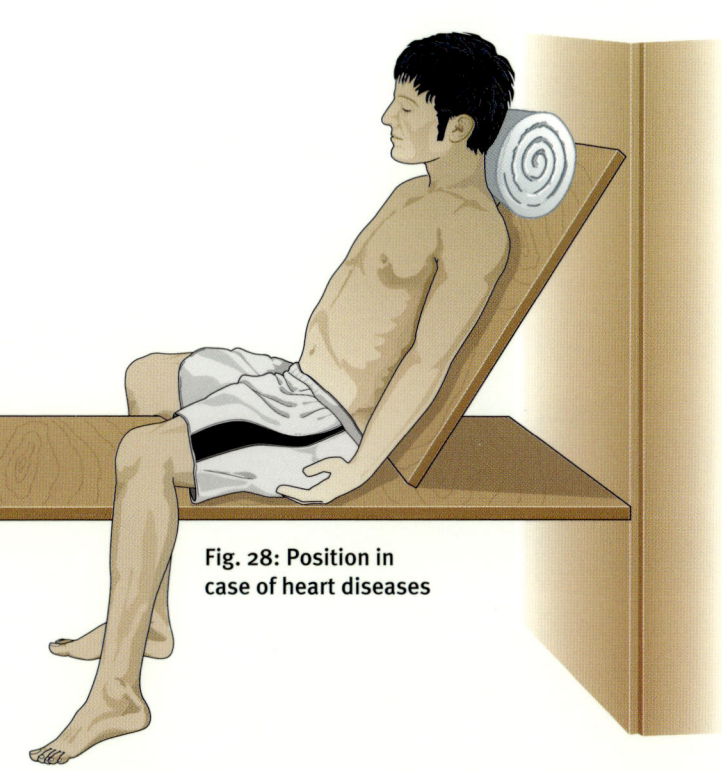

Fig. 28: Position in case of heart diseases

Blood Pressure Crisis
Synonyms: Cardiac Asthma, Hypertension

Causes
↘ Sudden high blood pressure (e.g. upper blood pressure of 160-250 mm Hg)

What else could it be?
↘ Chronic bronchitis or asthma: Underlying condition usually known, blood pressure not too high
↘ Heart attack: Blood pressure usually lower than normal

How to recognize?
↘ Breathing difficulties
↘ Chest pain
↘ Red, blushed face
↘ Prolonged exhalation phase
↘ Cough

What can happen?
↘ Weakening of the heart from overexertion, heart attack, or shock (life-threatening!)

What to do?
↘ Calm down
↘ Position to stabilize heart problems (see Fig. 28)

TIP If no medication is available but there is a blood measuring device, high-percentage alcohol can be administered in critical situations: It causes the widening of the vessels with a lower blood pressure. **Important:** Check blood pressure continually!

Shock
In case of shock, the supply of blood and oxygen to the body is diminished.

Causes
↘ Diseases with reduced heart strength
↘ Loss of blood and liquid (e.g. due to accident with bleeding, burn, diarrhea, vomiting)
↘ Allergic reaction
↘ Grave infection
↘ After rescue from water

What else could it be?
↘ All conditions like the ones mentioned above, but with less pronounced problems

How to recognize?
↘ Indicators for decreased heart strength (Page 23)
↘ Indicators for dehydration (Page 19)
↘ Low blood pressure, rapid pulse
↘ Cold sweat
↘ Paleness
↘ Confusion
↘ Fatigue, even unconsciousness
↘ Nausea, vomiting
↘ Fever or low body temperature

What can happen?
↘ Circulatory collapse (life-threatening! Refer to Page 7 and on)
↘ Impaired consciousness (life-threatening! Refer to Page 7 and on)

What to do?
- In case of decreased heart strength: Heart disease position (see Fig. 28)
- In case of all other causes: Positioning for someone in shock (Fig. 29)
- In case of bleeding: Stop bleeding, apply pressure bandage (Page 13)
- In case of allergic reaction: Stop contact with allergens
- In case of insect sting/bite: Cool the area

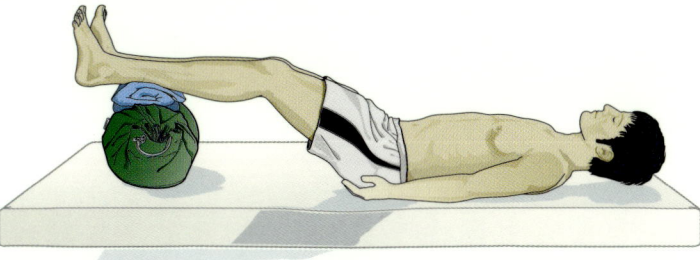

Fig. 29: Position for someone in shock

 TIP Shock prophylaxis in case of burns, diarrhea, or vomiting: Make sure sufficient liquid is ingested, perhaps apply fluid intravenously under the skin (Page 80).

Obstruction of Blood Vessels
Clots may cause the obstruction of vessels in veins or arteries (thrombosis or embolism).

Causes
Formation of a blood clot because of ...
- Slow circulation due to decreased mobility
- Slow circulation due to swelling after injury
- Heart arrhythmia

What else could it be?
- Swelling without obstruction of blood vessels: Injury, insect sting/bite
- Swelling of both calfs: Decreased heart strength

How to recognize?
- Vein and artery obstruction: Usually on one side only in one of the lower legs
- Vein obstruction: One-sided swelling, reddening, warming, sensation of heaviness
- Artery obstruction: Sudden and strong one-sided pain, paleness, coolness, impaired sensitivity (Page 21)

What can happen?
- Vein obstruction: Usually benign development
- Artery obstruction:
  - Dying of muscle tissue (amputation!)
  - Damage to inner organs (shock, life-threatening!)
- Rare: Blood clots dissolve or get relocated (pulmonary embolism, stroke)

What to do in case of vein obstruction?
- Raise limb
- Exercise
- Cold compresses

What to do in case of artery obstruction?
- Lower limb, soften position
- Immobilization: Absolutely no movement – lay the patient down and remove clothing (use scissors if need be). Do not let patient not get up, not even to urinate!
- Do not warm or cool!

> ⚠ Obstructions of the arteries are always life-threatening; the same is true for complications during a vein obstruction (e.g. pulmonary embolism). In such cases, it is very important to have radio-assisted consultation available! Sufficient prevention is **important**: In case of diminished physical activity (e.g. disease, rest after accident), perform regular exercises. In case of known thrombosis predilection, have thrombosis bandages fitted. Consult with your family doctor whether to bring along heparin.

Rib Concussion and Broken Rib after an Accident

Causes
- Fall

How to recognize?
- Visible injury at the chest
- Pressure pain while examining
- Intense pain when coughing and breathing deeply
- In case of several affected ribs: while inhaling, the chest of the affected side moves inside (paradoxic breathing)

What can happen?
- Injury of inner organs with bleeding and shock (Page 41)
- Pneumothorax (Page 16)
- Pneumonia (Page 38)

What else could it be?
- Coronary syndrome, heart attack: No pressure pain, no increased pain when inhaling and coughing
- Inflammation

What to do?
- If possible, discard pneumothorax: Examine (Page 24)
- Decrease pain by positioning onto the affected side (Fig. 30)
- Provide pain killers: Coughing and deep inhalation should be possible without problems

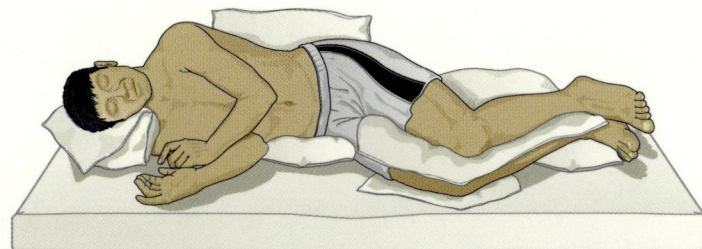

Fig. 30: Lateral position in case of rib concussion or broken rib.

Guiding Symptom – Abdominal Pain

Diseases of the abdomen can have many causes; they are usually benign and can be treated with items available on board. In case of serious abdominal illness, it is important to recognize the warning signs, which may indicate that rapid medical assistance is necessary. Indicators for harmless and serious causes for abdominal pain are:

Harmless Causes:
- Simple stomach infection
- Infection of the urinary tract

Serious Causes:
- Intestinal obstruction
- Appendicitis
- Gall bladder infection
- Withholding urine
- Renal colic
- Pyelitis

Warning Signs
- Bad general state
- Hard abdomen
- Abdominal pressure pain
- Spherical, inflated abdomen
- High fever
- Flank pain
- Rest position
- Protrusion/swelling with warming; probably pain in the groin, testicular or navel area
- Yellow discoloration of eyes and skin
- Continuous/increasing pain
- No noises from intestinal area
- Black stool
- Bloody vomit
- Novel bad reaction: coffee, fat, chocolate
- Rapid pulse
- Low blood pressure
- Rapid breath
- Signs of diminished heart strength

What to do?
- Immediately ask for medical consultation!

Await First Aid
- Good general state
- Little pain
- Soft abdomen
- Pain not continuous
- Concurrent vomiting and diarrhea
- Several persons with same symptoms
- Protrusion/swelling without warming and without pain in the groin, testicular or navel area
- Burning pain when urinating

What to do?
- Continue observation
- Treat with equipment and medication on board

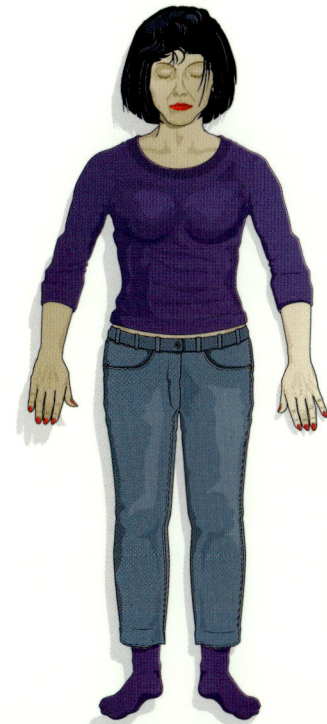

Fig. 31: Guiding Symptom – Abdominal Pain

Stomach Illnesses and Diseases

Harmless Stomach Illnesses

Causes
- Usually gastrointestinal infections
- Urinary tract infections due to damp/wet clothing
- More rare: Side effects of medication (e.g. antibiotics), sweetener, or alcohol

How to recognize?
Intestinal infection, side effects:
- Watery diarrhea (more than 3x per day) and/or vomiting
- In case of parasite infection (tropics): Stool often with blood clots
- Lively intestinal noises
- Possibly cramp-like pain without specific location

Urinary tract infection:
- Burning pain while urinating
- Possibly bloody urine
- Evaluate urine test strip (Page 29)

What can happen?
- Dehydration (Page 35)
- Missed warning signs
- Advancing urinary tract infection with kidney infection

What to do?
- Sufficient fluid intake
- Provide salty food
- Avoid further illness: Consider hygiene when handling patient

> **PLEASE NOTE**
> - Stomach illnesses up to five days usually do not require further treatment if the patient is in a generally good state of health.
> - In order to avoid infections, be careful to apply sufficient hygienic measures to food. Keep in mind this advice for tropical regions: *"Cook it, peel it—or forget it!"*

Serious Stomach Illnesses and Diseases

Causes
- **Intestinal obstruction:** After abdominal operations (even after years), with infections in the abdominal area, in case of strangulated hernias (groin, navel, scrotal hernias), tumors, or parasites, like worms (tropics)
- **Appendicitis:** No known risk factors
- **Gall bladder infection:** Mainly in case of kidney stone disease
- **Renal colic:** Due to kidney stones that reach the excretory urinary tract
- **Pyelitis:** Mainly due to "ascending" urinary tract infection
- **Urine retention:** Mainly in the case of males, usually with enlarged prostate; also in case of slipped disc

How to recognize?
- **General indications for a serious cause:** Fig. 31
- **Intestinal obstruction:** Swollen abdomen, probably hard, usually lively intestinal noises (Page 27); sometimes stool retention or stool-like vomit; pain without typical quadrant localization (see Fig. 23); possible quick deterioration of the general state
- **Strangulated hernia:** Swelling in the navel area, groin, testicles, or old scars from operations; possible development over time
- **Appendicitis:** Page 29
- **Gall bladder infection:** Pain mainly after greasy meals; yellowish discoloration of eyes and skin (usually only during developed stages); pain particularly in the right upper quadrant (see Fig. 23); sometimes radiation of pain into the right shoulder
- **Renal colic:** Starts with wave-like pain in one flank, radiating pain into the lower quadrant of the same side and groin, testicles, or labia (Page 28)
- **Pyelitis:** Pain in flank (Page 28), usually occurs prior to urinary tract infection (Page 29)
- **Urine retention:** Pain between the two upper quadrants (Fig. 23)

What else could it be?
- **Heart attack:** New cardiac arrhythmias; if available, perform troponin test (Page 27) — equipment onboard is not sufficient to contain this condition
- **Gynecological disease:** Equipment on board is not sufficient to contain this condition
- **Gastric ulcer:** Primarily pain, less "warning indicators"

What can happen?
- Dehydration (Page 35)
- Peritonitis or infection of the entire body (sepsis) with shock (Page 41, life-threatening!)

What to do?
- **In case of intestinal obstruction, appendicitis or gall bladder infection:** Do not eat (take medication with a small amount of water), rest, place in stable abdominal position (Fig. 32)
- **In case of strangulated hernia:** Try to push back the strangulated section; the muscles of the patient need to be relaxed while doing so: press your flat hand onto the protrusion and use the fingers of the other hand to try to massage the protrusion back through the opening. Do not permit patient to lift heavy items!
- **In case of pyelitis:** Drink plenty of fluids
- **In case of renal colic:** Drink plenty of fluids, move around; it is best to walk down stairs
- **In case of urine retention:** If possible, catheterize

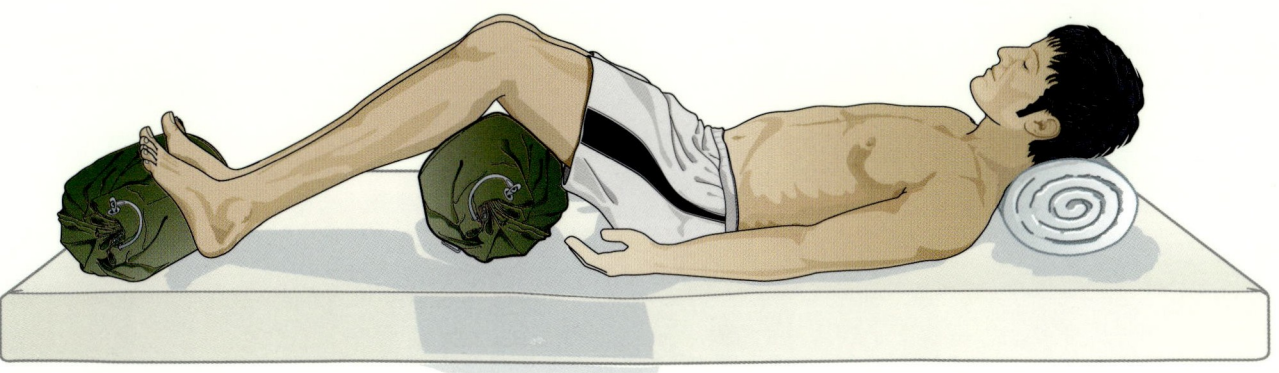

Fig. 32: Abdominal position

TAKE NOTE

- Normal stool evacuation does not preclude an intestinal obstruction.
- A sudden, but often only passing, decrease of pain is an indication of a perforation (rupture of a hollow organ).
- In case the massage of an hernia back into the body is successful, there is no necessity for an urgent operation.
- In case of a known enlargement of the prostate or prior cases of urine retention, it makes sense to previously learn the catheterization of the bladder (family doctor) and to bring along the corresponding equipment.

 TIP It makes no sense to remove the appendix beforehand—even if the planned journey is far away from any medical help for an extended period of time! Every operation in the abdominal area means a higher risk for an abdominal obstruction.

Effects of Heat, Cold, or Water

The effects of heat, cold and water are common on board and may become life-threatening:
- Drowning • Sunlight incidence
- Hypothermia • Burns • Frostbite

Drowning

Immersion in water with resulting respiratory problems, particularly due to a panic reaction. Quickly appearing symptoms of hypothermia is dangerous.

Causes
- Fall into water: Accident, sudden unconsciousness
- While in the water: Diving, sudden illness

How to recognize?
- Panic reaction

What can happen?
In the water:
- Due to panic reaction: Swallowing or breathing in water, high breathing frequency, increase of pulse and blood pressure
- In case of pre-existing conditions, particularly of the heart: Immediate death (e.g. due to cardiac arrest or arrhythmia)
- Breathing in sea spray: With prolonged time in the water, larger quantities are a possibility
- In case of sudden unconsciousness: Immediate asphyxiation is possible
- The affected person is quickly unable to assist with his or her rescue, as their strength and coordination are impaired

During the rescue:
- Danger of vomiting: Stomach may be full of swallowed water
- Aspiration: Stomach content gets into the breathing passages during the rescue or due to diminished reflexes. Possible results: Complete obstruction of the breathing passages (starting on Page 14) and pneumonia
- Accumulation of water in the lung or pulmonary edema: Cause is often not breathed-in water, but heart insufficiency after a drowning accident
- Death during rescue: Due to the diminished water pressure during the rescue, the blood pressure plummets, causing shock or unconsciousness (Page 7)

What to do?
- Rules for affected person: Move very little, leave on clothing, lay in fetal position (Fig. 33); in case of several persons in the water, remain close together
- Rescue: If possible, place in horizontal position; diminished risk of death during rescue
- If not possible (as in most cases): Rescue as quickly as possible, place in immediate shock position on board (see Fig. 29), check vital parameters, resuscitate if required (Page 9)

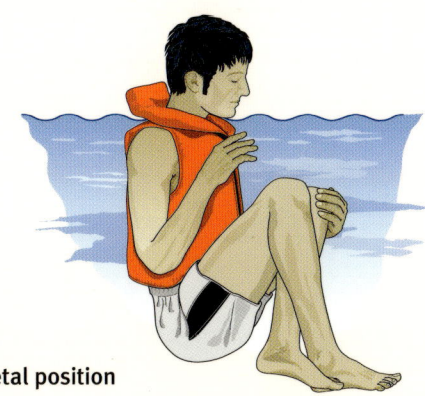

Fig. 33: Fetal position

Whether or not a strong member of the crew leaves the vessel during a rescue is always a personal decision. The endangering of more people must always be avoided!

Hypothermia

Hypothermia means the lowering of the body's temperature to below 36 ºC, e.g. due to an increased loss of body heat in the water; it depends on the circumstances, such as water and outer temperature, and also on individual factors such as clothing, body type or prior illnesses. Typical signs, even during the early stages, are impaired reactions, strength and coordination, with impaired vital parameters ensuing quickly.

TAKE NOTE

- Radio-assisted consultation is required after State II without sign of improvement.
- Children lose body heat more quickly; however, the possibility of a complete recovery is better.
- It is not necessary to measure the body temperature; treatment is based solely on the symptoms.
- Never provide alcohol to "warm up" — it increases the loss of body heat!
- No active heating, no hot compresses, no close body contact!
- A defibrillation in case of severe hypothermia may not be successful — nevertheless apply in case of emergency!

How to recognize?	What to do?
Stage I	**Stage I**
• Agitation stage: with shivering • Body temperature 96.8–91.4ºF (36-33ºC)	• Keep patient warm, provide warm beverages • Allow patient to move just a little (putting on and off clothes) • Signs of improvement: Shivering stops, patient is awake or easy to wake up
Stage II	**Stage II**
• Exhaustion Stage: no shivering; reflexes, strength, and coordination noticeably diminished • Decreasing breathing frequency • Body temperature 91.4–86ºF (33-30ºC) • Impaired consciousness	• Keep warm, provide small amounts of warm beverage • Do not allow to move, remove clothing with scissors • Observe constantly • Signs of improvement: Shivering
Stage III	**Stage III and IV**

• Paralysis Stage: Reflexes, strength, and coordination strongly diminished
• Cardiac arrhythmias very likely
• Body temperature lower than 86ºF (30ºC)
	• No pulse, no breathing
	  ↘ resuscitation (Page 9)
	• Existing pulse, no breathing
	  ↘ artificial respiration (Page 9)
	• Pulse and breathing present
	  ↘ stable lateral position (Page 8)
	• Check vital parameters regularly (Page 6)

Stage IV	
Apparent Death: No noticeable vital parameters	

> If the patient is shivering, then there is no danger!

Frostbite

In case of frostbite on board, individual body parts are affected, mostly the face, hands, and feet.

Causes
- Cold affecting body with reduced circulation due to wet and constricting clothing

How to recognize
- Early phase: feeling cold, pain, swelling, red skin
- Later: increasing pain and feeling of cold decrease, dark-red and violet skin color, hard tissue
- Late phase: no pain, white discoloration of the skin

What can happen?
- With decreasing pain, frostbite is not paid attention to or treated
- Large area with tissue damage, with ensuing infection and organ damage
- Compartment syndrome: Due to swelling, there is a higher pressure in the tissue, decreased circulation, and, thus, damage of nerves and organs (Page 56)

What to do?
- The affected person must actively move—moving passively is not going to help!
- Gradual warming by: Water bath or warm compresses 95–104°F (35–40°C)
- Avoid pressure due to blankets
- Do not rub or massage — tissue damage may be increased!

> **PLEASE NOTE**
>
> Frostbite can become life-threatening if left untreated. As a precautionary measure, warm, dry, and unrestricting clothing should always be worn; exposed parts such as the nose, ears, toes, or fingers should always be well-protected.

Solar Radiation

At sea, the intensity of the sun´s rays is several times higher due to the reflections; it is common to underestimate them because of the cooling wind.

Causes
- **Sunburn:** Skin reaction after too much exposure to the sun.
- **Sunstroke/Insolation:** Swelling of the brain after too much exposure to the sun, especially if the head is unprotected (e.g. not wearing a hat).
- **Heat exhaustion:** Dehydration in case of insufficient water intake.
- **Heat stroke:** Warming with insufficient heat release (tight clothing).

How to recognize?
- **Sunburn:** Typical skin changes (burns up to grade IIA)
- **Sunstroke:** Strong headache, nausea, impaired consciousness leading to coma, muscle cramps

- **Heat exhaustion:** Exhaustion, rapid pulse, low blood pressure, headaches, paleness. More rare: cramps and muscle pain
- **Heat stroke:** Exhaustion, rapid pulse, low blood pressure, impaired consciousness, raised body temperature, reddish skin

What else could it be?
- Seasickness (Page 74)
- Hypothermia (Page 49)
- Impaired consciousness (Page 33)

What can happen?
- Life-threatening impaired consciousness

What to do
- **Always:** Drink plenty of water and avoid going out in the sun or, if you have to, cover up.
- **Sunburn:** See below (burns)
- **Sunstroke:** Rest with upper body raised and cold compresses; in case of mild symptoms, cool the head only.
- **Heat exhaustion:** In case of diminished heart strength, lay to avoid going into shock.
- **Heat stroke:** Rest with upper body raised and cold compresses.

PLEASE NOTE

Too much solar radiation can be life-threatening if left untreated. As a precautionary measure, drink a lot of fluids (no alcohol!), keep in the shade, and wear adequate clothing. Remember: Sun lotion protects only against sunburn!

Burn Wounds

Burn wounds are not among the most common injuries when on board a sea-going vessel; however, they are painful and can become infected, so they should be treated with diligence.

Causes
Heat incidence due to …
- open fire and hot surfaces
- solar radiation
- mechanical friction (e.g. ropes)

How to recognize?
Divided according to grade of burn and extension.

Burn grades:
- I°: Superficial, reddening, pain
- II°A: Reddening, blisters, pain
- II°B: Pink-white, blisters, little pain
- III°: White, leather-like, no pain
- IV°: Blackening

Extension:
There is an immediate threat to life if burns extend over more than 15 percent of the body. The percentage of burn wounds with respect to the body's area is important for the treatment. It can be quickly determined using the one percent rule (Fig. 34) or the rule of nine (Fig. 35).

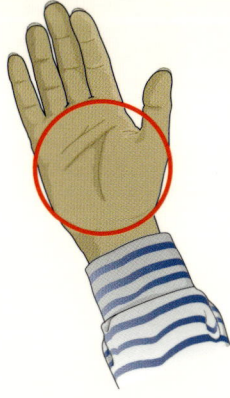

Fig. 34: One percent-rule to determine the extent of burn injuries

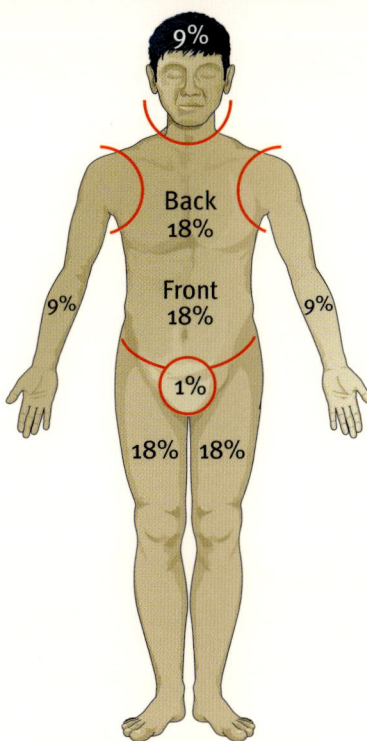

Fig. 35: Rule of nine-percent to determine the extent of burn wounds.

The inner hand surface without the fingers of the affected person (red circle) corresponds to about 1% of the body's surface area (this applies to all ages).

9%: One arm, head
18%: One leg, front upper body, rear upper body
1%: Genital area

What can happen?
⇘ Misjudgment of seriousness in case of only little pain from grade II°B and higher
⇘ Burn sickness: Threat to life due to loss of liquid and tissue dying off.
⇘ Smoke inhalation: Indicators are burnt eyebrows, eyelashes, or nostril hairs, soot around the nostrils, hoarseness, difficulty swallowing. Danger: There can be major breathing difficulties even hours later.

What to do?
First measures
⇘ Stop further burning: Put out with water, cover flames with blanket, even jump into the water
⇘ Cooling: Every 15 minutes with lukewarm water or cool rag (no ice!); if possible, only the affected area
⇘ End cooling if the patient feels cold
⇘ Next, protect against getting cold (rescue blanket)

Further Treatment on Land
⇘ Cover wound with sterile dressing
⇘ If necessary, provide painkillers
⇘ See a doctor!

PLEASE NOTE
Burn injuries and burn shock are dangerous and even under the best of circumstances in a hospital they are often problematic.

Do not cool if more than 30% of the body is affected – it increases the risk of infection.

Further treatment if no help available
- Carefully clean wounds: With boiled water, disinfectant or infusion fluid (see Fig. 52)
- Clean instruments (Page 64)
- Remove dirt with tweezers
- Do not open blisters!
- Keep burn wounds moistened: Apply thin, sterile layer of burn balm or fat (with a wooden spatula) and cover with greased gauze
- Protect burn wounds: Cover with dressing, affix loosely with gauze bandage
- Watch for signs of infection (Page 19)
- Watch for sufficient fluid intake
- Avoid infections: Change dressing every 24 hours; remove dead skin with scalpel (source of infection)

Burns can be life-threatening if left untreated. It is necessary to get radio-assisted help. The following cases require a rapid medical assistance, if necessary by evacuation:

- I° to II°B: In cases where more than 10% (adults) or 5% (children) of body area are affected
- III°: In cases where more than 2% of children's or adult's area are affected
- If hands, face, genitals, or large articulations are affected
- In cases of smoke inhalation

Required Supplies
- Examination gloves
- Rinsing fluid, sterile is best (e.g. infusion fluid); rinsing cannules
- Tweezers, scalpel
- Wooden spatula
- Gauze wound dressings, covered wound dressings (non-stick), gauze bandages
  Important: The side of aluminum-covered wound dressings goes onto the wound.
- Burn ointment: See medication (Page 70)

 Burn wounds can easily get infected. Keep things clean and disinfect your hands and instruments regularly!

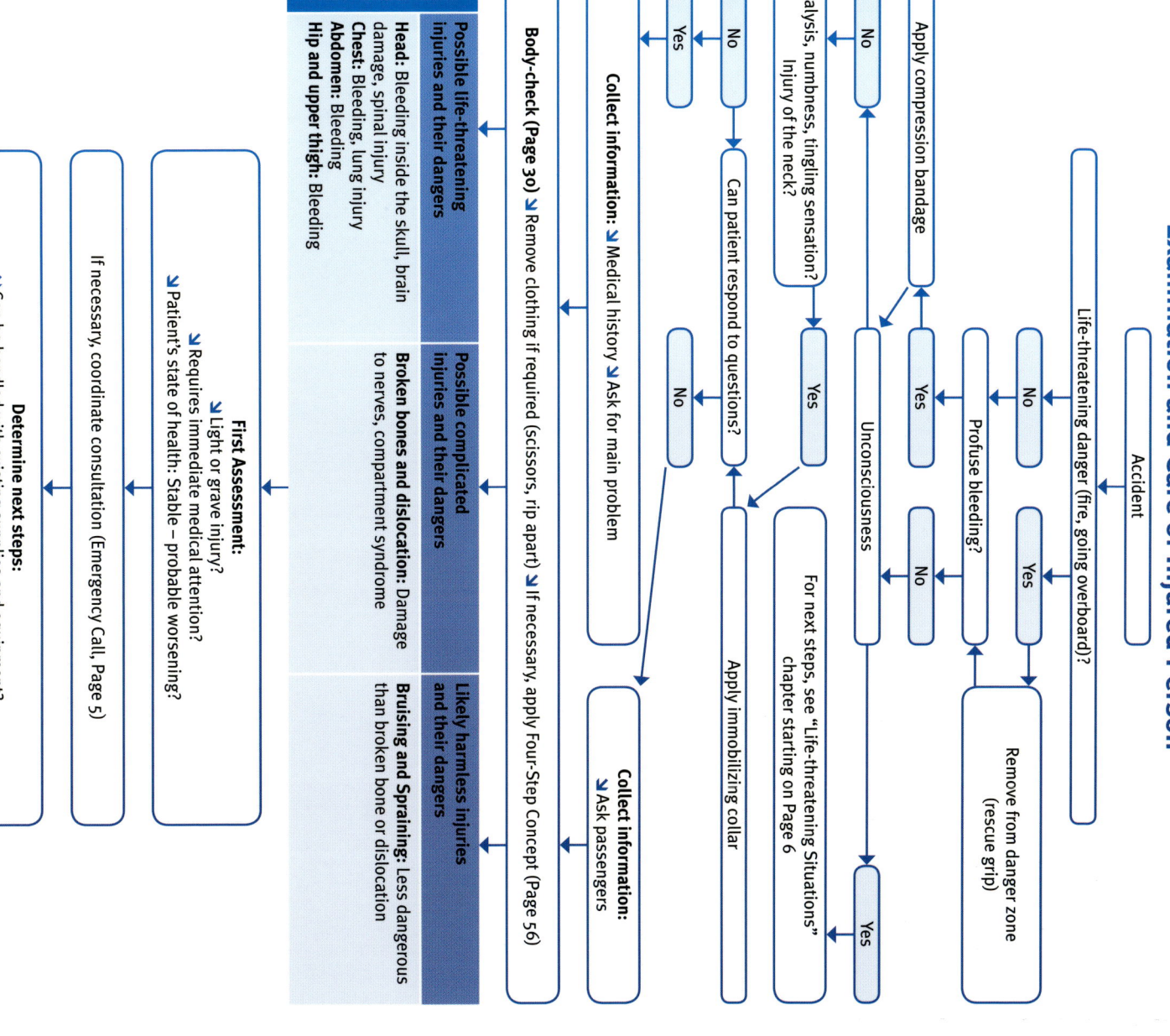

Compact Lexicon of Orthopedic and Surgical Terms
Top extremities: Arms
Lower extremities: Legs
Neutral position: Position with relaxed extremities
Contusion: Bruising of skin, muscles, bones, or organs; the skin can remain undamaged
Sprain/Distortion: Momentary separation of the areas of an articulation
Dislocation: Ongoing separation of areas of an articulation
Shifting/dislocation: Change of position after dislocation or broken bone
Position correction: Intent to correct a shift or to achieve a painless position
Broken bone (fracture): Separation of a bone

Among the most important illnesses and injuries of the locomotor system on board are:
- Bruises
- Sprains
- Dislocation
- Fractures

A definitive distinction is often not possible. Water sports mainly affect:
- Head
- Wrist
- Ribs
- Finger
- Ankle
- Lower arm

In case of a stronger impact (e.g. fall, getting hit by the boom), the following body parts may be affected:
- Upper arm
- Collarbone
- Lower arm
- Spine
- Shoulder (mostly dislocations)
- Lower leg

Injuries to the upper thigh and the hip are rather rare. Some of the injuries can be taken care of with only a few measures; others require a high degree of medical knowledge and training.

The basic care of injuries to the locomotor system are always the same; only sprains and contortions or fractures may require a more complex approach.

How to recognize?
- Pain
- Swelling
- Impaired mobility
- In case of sprains and fractures: Bad positioning
- In case of fracture: Certain signs for broken bones include . . .
  - Friction between bone
  - Wrong position of axis
  - Abnormal mobility
  - Visibly broken bone
  - Open fracture: Visible bone parts, wound in the area of fracture
  - "Almost certain" sign of fracture: Compression pain (Page 30, body-check)
- In case of fractures: Uncertain signs for broken bones include . . .
  - Pain
  - Swelling
  - Change of shape
  - Diminished mobility
  - Exposed bone without visible fracture

INJURIES OF THE LOCOMOTOR SYSTEM

What can happen?
Additional possible injuries:
- Sprained or torn ligament
- Bleeding into the muscle tissue: Bruise, hematoma
- Profuse bleeding in case of injuries to the chest, hip, thigh, and inner organs
- Nerve and cartilage damage
- Long-lasting impairment after major accidents
- Compartment syndrome

> ⚠️ **Compartment Syndrome**
> Complications after injuries, often to the lower arm and thigh.
> **How to recognize?** Hard swelling of the injured area, decreasing sensitivity (Page 21) behind the injury, nail test takes fairly long (Page 23).
> **What can happen?** Due to the increasing swelling, there is a diminished circulation and a possible damage to nerves and muscles. The necrosis of muscle tissue can cause damage to other organs (particularly the kidneys).
> **What to do?** A compartment syndrome is life-threatening! Apply the Four-Step Concept without compression and quickly get professional help (radio-assisted help!).

What to do after an Accident?
It is important to avoid swelling and pain by icing, cooling, and immobilizing the affected area.

Basic treatment
- Examine and care for injured person (Page 54)
- Examine the injured person: Body-check (Page 30)
- Proceed according to the Four-Step Concept (see sidebar)
- In case of indications that the head or spine are affected: Apply immobilizing collar (Page 59)

> **FOUR-STEP Concept**
> - **Rest:** Immobilize affected body part, stabilize if required (stabilizing splint, Page 60)
> - **Ice:** Cool as quickly as possible for 30-45 minutes, e.g. with self-cooling aggregates
> - **Compression:** Wrap with bandages
> - **Raise limb:** Several times per day after the accident

Special Characteristics in case of Sprains and Fractures
- Change of position
- Stabilization and immobilization

Change of Position
Prior to any change of position, apply the basic care. Required conditions for a change of position:
- Indications for a fracture or sprain
- Stabilization without change of position does not cause diminishing pain
- Complications: Indications of damage nerves or blood vessels
- No professional care available for 5-10 hours
- The patient agrees
- The measure is recommended via radio-assisted consultation

Purposes
- Reduce pain
- Maintain blood flow
- Avoid tissue and nerve damage

What can happen?
- After a change of position, a renewed dislocation is possible.
- Due to compression (such as increasing swelling), a compartment syndrome is possible.
- The intention to make a change of position can cause tissue, nerve, or blood vessel damage — consider before performing it!

Indications
- Change of position and immobilization are painful and technically difficult.
- Novices can only perform the change of position of the ankle, lower leg, lower arm, and finger bones.
- After a successful change of position, professional care is still necessary.

How to do?
- Principle: Pull and counter-pull along the long axis of the affected limb.
- A successful change of position is often audible and leads to diminished pain.
- Maintain the pull until the change of position is achieved (stabilization).
- Regularly check pulse, and perform nail test (Page 23) and sensitivity test (Page 21).

Change of Position of the Lower Arm
- Thumb and lower arm should form a straight line: Angle the hand towards the side of the pinky (Fig. 36).
- The hand is always fixed using a thick bandage in the "boxing glove" position.
- Pull at the hand at the thumb side, e.g. with a line around a winch.

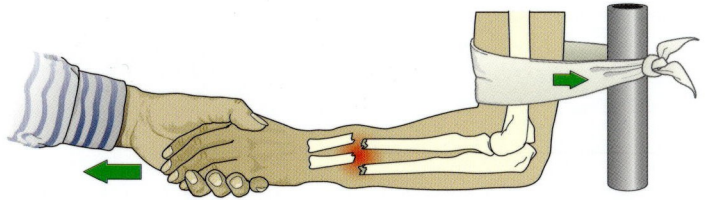
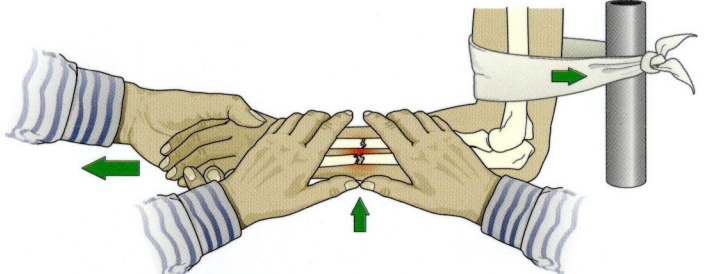

Fig. 36: Change of Position of the Lower Arm

IMPORTANT

The pulse should be present behind the splinted area or the bandage. Indicators of a worsening condition are a pale or blue discolored skin and tingling or absence of sensitivity. Perform often:
- Feel the pulse (Page 23)
- Check sensitivity (Page 21)

In case of deteriorating conditions, loosen constricting bandages or splints if possible.

Change of Position at the Ankle
- One hand holds the outer ankle and steadily pulls at the foot.
- The other hand holds the leg at the inner ankle and pushes against it.
- After successful change of position: Stabilize foot in a 90-degree position to the lower leg (Fig. 38).

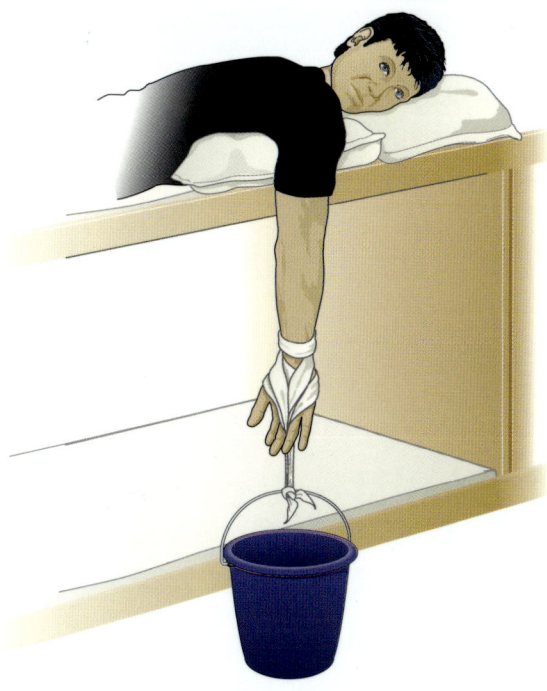

Fig. 37: Change of position in case of shoulder dislocation

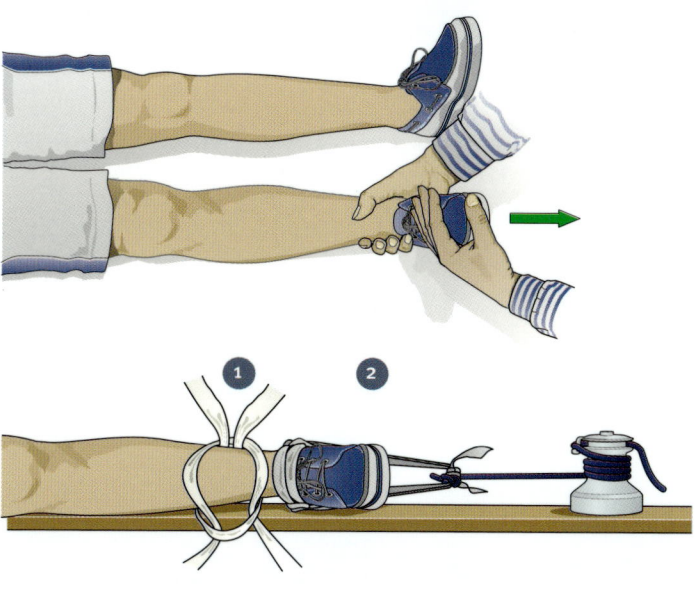

Fig. 38: Change of position at the ankle

Change of Position in case of Shoulder Dislocation
- Turn the arm 45 degrees to the outside (Fig. 37)
- Increase the weight in the bucket continuously until reaching some 7 kg, or 15 lbs.
- Helpers can shift the pull-point towards the head
- To immobilize the shoulder, also bandage the upper arm to the torso

Some people are prone to shoulder dislocations; in these cases, it is advisable to practice the change of position and immobilization beforehand.

Stabilization and Immobilization
Alternatives for stabilization (prepare beforehand):
- Immobilizing collar: To stabilize the neck
- Stabilizing splint: Sufficient stabilization possible
- Cast splint: Optimal stabilization; needs practice
- Inflatable splint: Can damage tissue; use only temporarily (during transport)
- Alternatives: Rolled-up newspaper, cushion, boards, or rudder/paddle (see Fig. 41)

Apply immobilizing collar

The immobilizing collar serves the purpose of stabilizing the neck where the spine may have been damaged. The collar should be put on prior to the rescue. Examples of an immobilizing collar is the Stifneck®; it is available in adult and children sizes. If the collar is set too large, it may lead to over-stretching; if set too small, it may lead to an instability of the cervical spine — practice its use before starting your trip.

> **IMPORTANT**
>
> Immobilization is not complete — avoid all unnecessary movements. Do not remove collar until an x-ray has been taken to confirm or exclude injury. A soft neck collar (e.g. rolled newspaper/foam splint) is not an alternative!

How to do?

- Set collar size: Measure the distance between shoulders and chin and set the appropriate size (Fig. 39: 1–3)
- Lock the chosen size (4)
- Put on:
  - From below the chin, push up the chin rest (5). In case of reclining patients, first pull the back of the collar under the neck and then put on chin rest.
  - Always note: Head must be looking straight forward (neutral position); slight pull to the top is best (5).
- Fixation: Hold the frontal part, pull tight the rear section (6).

> **IMPORTANT**
>
> If possible, always stabilize/immobilize neighboring articulations: In case of an injured lower arm, the hand and elbow is immobilized; a broken thigh is affixed to the other thigh.

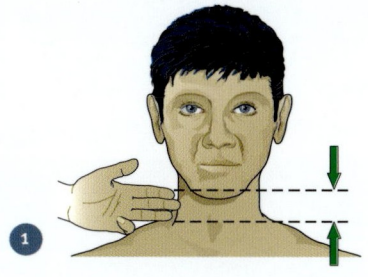
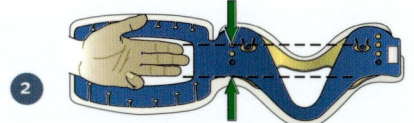
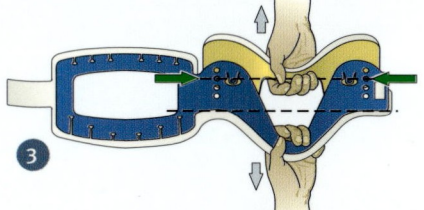
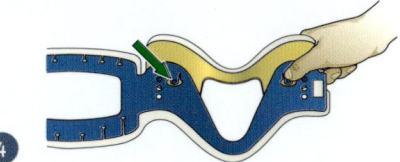
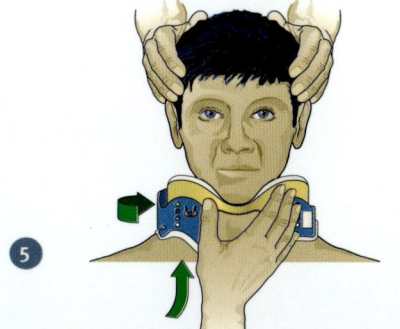
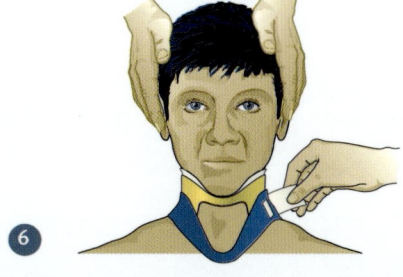

Fig. 39: Putting on immobilizing collar

Applying a Stabilizing Splint

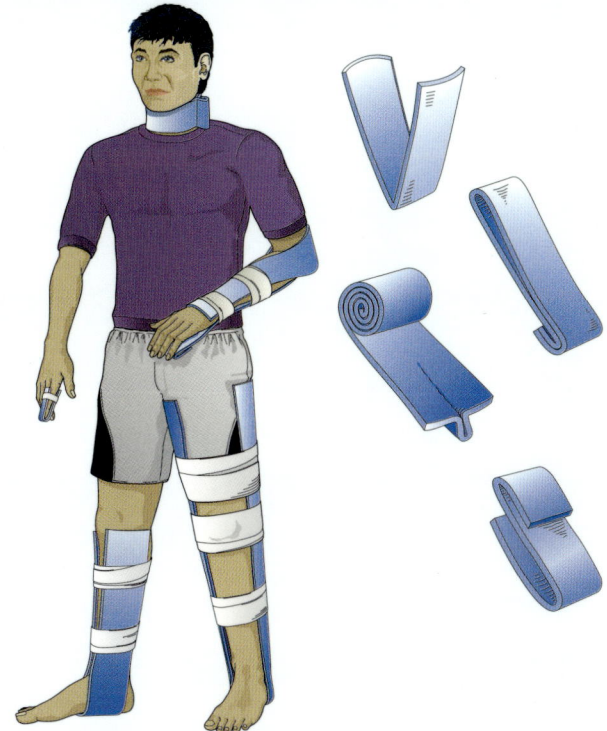

Fig. 40: Put on splint. Sections of the splint may be cut off.

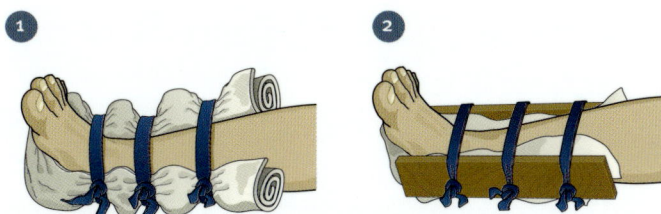

Fig. 41: Stabilizing the ankle. Splint with ..
❶ rolled-up towel/blanket or newspaper
❷ boards

Immobilizing the Knee and Lower Leg
- Cushion the heel to avoid pressure marks
- If using splints, put the foot into a 90-degree position to the lower leg

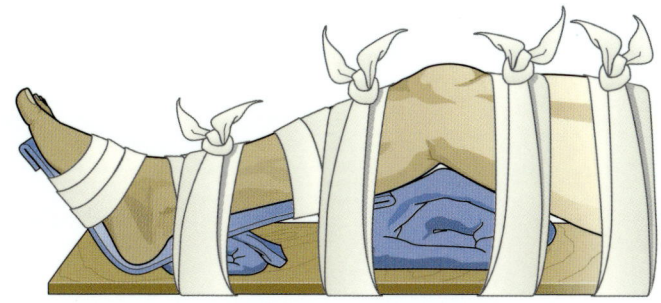

Fig. 42: Immobilization of knee and lower leg

Immobilizing the Fingers, Hand, and Lower Arm

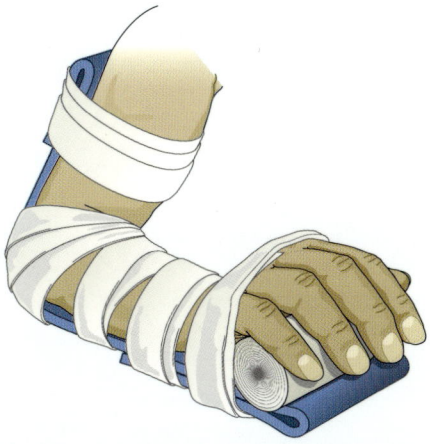

Fig. 43: Immobilization of fingers, hand, and lower arm

Immobilization in Case of Fractured Rib or Collarbone

Use a triangular cloth (Fig. 44) on the side with the fracture; in case of fractured rib, also fixate the arm with wide bandages to the torso (Fig. 45). In case of acute breathing problems, see Page 39.

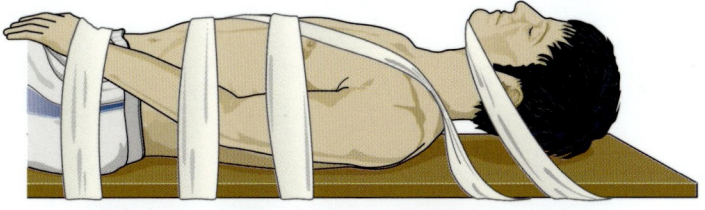

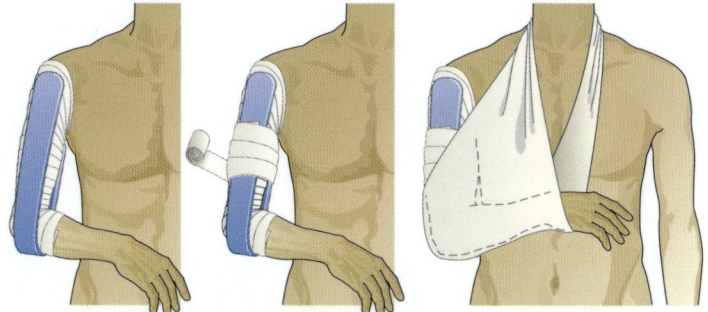

Fig. 44: Immobilization of upper arm, elbow, and shoulder

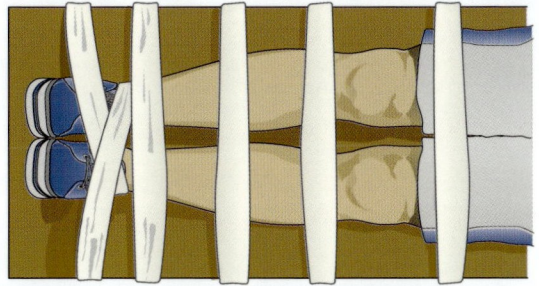

Fig. 46: Stabilizing and immobilizing of hip and spine

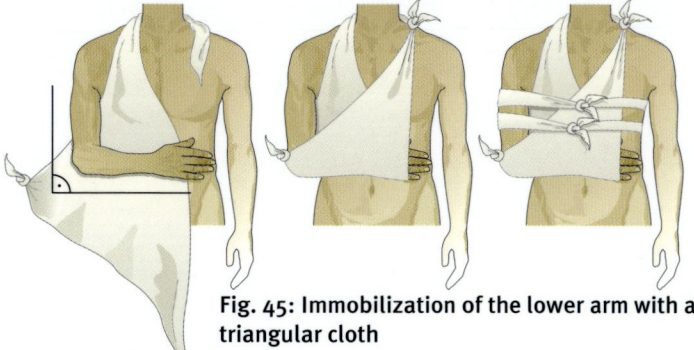

Fig. 45: Immobilization of the lower arm with a triangular cloth

Immobilizing the Hip and Spine

- In case of hip or spine fractures, immobilize the entire body (e.g. on cockpit grating or wooden board; Fig. 46)
- Bandage the legs (blanket, rope)
- Blanket to cushion; place between the legs
- Affix the feet facing towards the inside

Taking Care of Open Fractures

- If Help is available within 10 hours:
  - In case of heavy soiling: Rinse, infusion fluid is best; alternatively use previously boiled water (see Fig. 51 and 52)
  - Cover with sterile bandages
- If no Help is available within 10 hours:
  - Remove foreign objects and dead tissue (tweezers and scalpel) – keep everything clean!
  - Rinse, infusion fluid is best; alternatively with previously boiled water (see Fig. 51 and 52)
  - Try change of position, immobilize
  - Clean wound again
  - You might cover the wound with skin and wound dressing
  Important: Do not close the wound with a clip or with stitches!

 Open fractures are prone to infections and must always be treated professionally!

Other Injuries

Eye Irritation and Inflammation
Causes: Often due to wind and strong sunlight, rarely due to inflammation
How to recognize? Reddening, tears, itching; in case of infection: pus

> In case of infection, use regular rinses (eye rinse). Only use antibiotic ointments when there are indications of a bacterial infection. In case of conjunctivitis, consult with your family doctor prior to the trip.

Foreign Object in the Eye
Causes: Sand, insects, sea water, paint
How to recognize? Pain, tears
Examination: Open eyes, illuminated from the side. If insufficient: evert eyelid (Fig. 48)

> The sensation of having a foreign object in the eye often persists after removing it. If such a sensation persists for more than 12 hours or there is a more serious eye injury, contact a doctor under all circumstances!

Eye Injury
Causes: Tool, glass, or metal shard
How to recognize? Usually by the accident's features and development, might be difficult: Bleeding, altered pupil shape, decreased visual ability

What to do in case of inflammation and injuries of the eye?
Simple cases (uncomplicated irritation or inflammation, uncomplicated foreign objects):
- Rinse with eye bath or water bottle (Fig. 47)
- Loose foreign object: Remove with swab

Complicated cases (stuck foreign object, injury)
- Get medical consultation
- Stuck foreign object: If a doctor cannot be reached in the foreseeable future, try to remove the foreign object with a blunt object. Metal particles may be moved using a magnet
- Avoid any pressure and eye movement, clean eye, and bandage both eyes; get medical help as quickly as possible

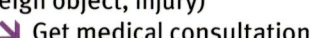
Fig. 47: Eye bath

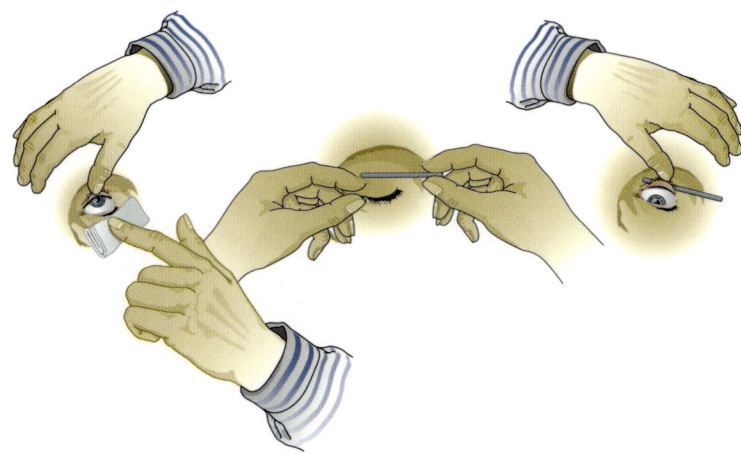
Fig. 48: Examining and everting the eyelid

Nosebleed

Nosebleeds are usually harmless and the source of blood is usually the frontal part of the nose.
Cause: Injury

What to do?
- Press nasal wings together for about 15 minutes
- Place head forwards.
- Put something cold onto the back of the neck (e.g. towel, cooling pack).
- If possible, take blood pressure.
- Not sufficient? Moisten rolled-up tissue with nose-drops (Page 68), insert into nostril, and continue pressing together.
- Not sufficient? The source of bleeding may be further in the back and cannot be compressed using the fingers; patient might have to be evacuated.

Hematoma under the Finger- or Toenail

Hematomas are usually harmless and heal without further measures taken.
Cause: Injury, blow

What to do?
- First Aid: Use FOUR-STEP concept (Page 56)
- In case of pain due to increase of swelling: Release pressure with a bent paper-clip heated over an open flame (fig. 49)
- Disinfect nail, cover loosely, keep dry

Fishhook Injury
What to do?

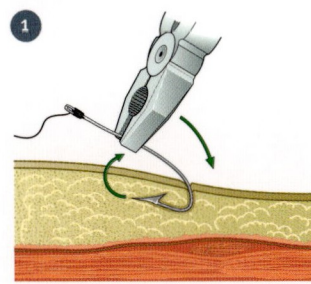

❶ Push hook all the way through the skin (do not pull out!).

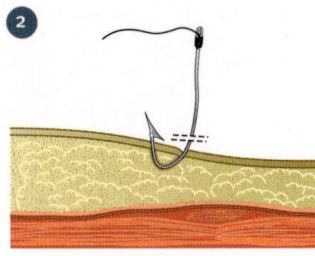

❷ Hold the tip of the hook with pliers and cut through it at the point where it enters the skin.

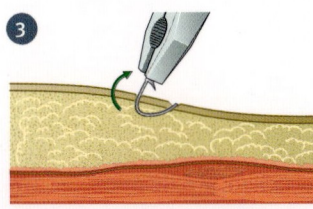

❸ Remove tip and rest of the hook and continue with basic wound care (Page 64).

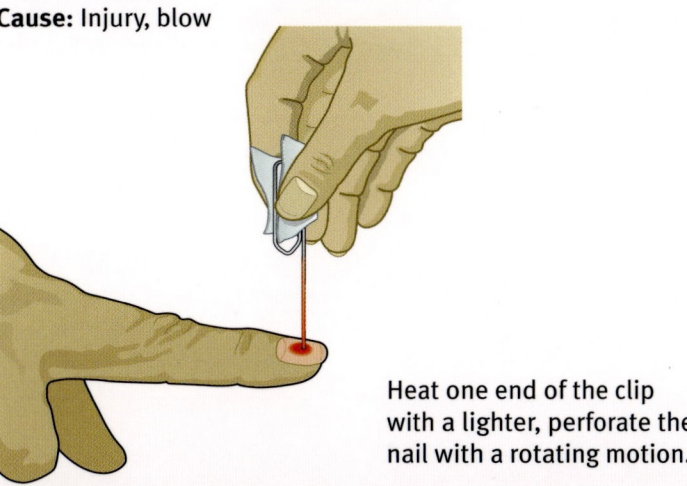

Heat one end of the clip with a lighter, perforate the nail with a rotating motion.

Fig. 49: Pressure release at nail

Fig. 50: Removing fishhook

Wound Care

The skin acts as a barrier against germs and diseases. Every wound means there is a disturbance of this function. In order to avoid complications, wounds should be cared for with diligence. Usually, cleaning the wound and applying a band aid is sufficient. Larger wounds require a more complex method. A wound closes in about ten days. During this time, there is the possibility of an infection. Rinsing a wound can effectively prevent this.

Gauze bandages are available as ready-to-use packs, including wound dressing. To affix the wound dressings, large and adhesive dressings are particularly suitable. It tends to slip or move less and can be affixed to any part of the body.

Materials Needed for Wound Care

- Waterproof band-aids of various sizes, blister band-aids
- Spray for superficial wounds and abrasions
- Strong adhesive tape roll (e.g. 2.5 x 500 cm)
- Gauze wound dressings
- Wound dressings with aluminum coating: for wounds with high likelihood of infection (e.g. burns, open fractures)
- To affix the wound dressings: Gauze bandages, adhesive dressing (with retention)
- For larger wounds: Rinsing cannula (see Fig. 51)
- To close the wound: Agraffe band-aid (Fig. 54), perhaps stitching material
- For problematic wounds (e.g. after a burn): Gauze wound dressings
- For squished fingers: Leather finger cot
- Instruments: Wound- and shard tweezers, razor, scalpel, bandage and wound scissors, cannula for foreign objects that are deeply inserted under the skin
- Disinfectant, sterile swabs
- Examination gloves
- Office paperclip: To relieve hematomas under foot and finger nails (see Fig. 49)

Preparing for Wound Care

Clean the instruments before performing the wound care and proceed with diligence:
- Boil instruments in water for about 20 minutes or at least clean with disinfectant and a sterile swab.
- Clean and disinfect hands; wear examination gloves and sterilize
- Do not leave instruments at patient's side when leaving the area
- If instruments are soiled during the treatment (removing foreign object, pus): Clean with disinfectant and sterile swab or bandage.

IMPORTANT

Boiling in water does not provide a complete sterility of the instruments!

Basic Wound Care

- Remove foreign object with sterile swab or disinfected wound tweezers
- Rinse wound
- Disinfect wound
- Remove hair around the wound area with scissors or razor (danger of infection!)
- Change dressing daily; look for signs of infection (Page 19)

> **IMPORTANT**
>
> Always keep your own protection in mind—wear examining gloves when caring for wounds.

How to do? – Rinse wounds
- Rinse wound daily, more often if infected
- Utilize non-alcoholic disinfectant; alternatively, boiled water or drinking water
- To rinse the deeper sections of a wound: Rinsing cannule with flexible and blunt end (Fig. 51)
- Alternative rinsing method: Pouch with one corner cut off (Fig. 52)

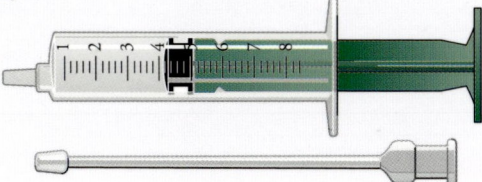

Fig. 51: Syringe and cannula rinsing for cleaning the wound

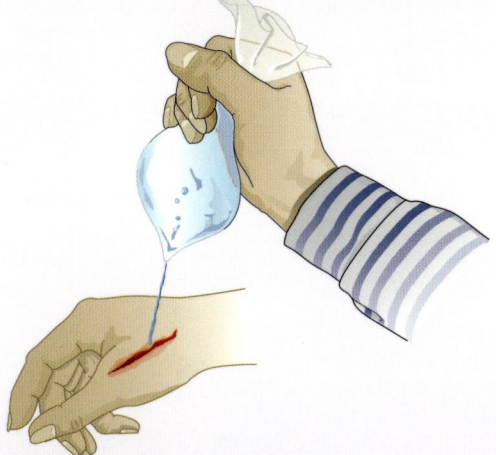

Fig. 52: Alternative to a rinsing cannula

Non-alcoholic disinfectants (e.g. Octenisept®) do not cause a burning sensation when touching the wound; thus, they are used for wound rinsing. Take note: Octenisept must be able to flow off after rinsing and must not be injected into closed-off pouches. **Alcoholic disinfectants** (e.g. Sterillium®) are particularly suitable for disinfection of the skin due to their fat-dissolving effect.

How to do? – Disinfect wounds
- Soak sterile swab with alcoholic disinfectant
- Clean the area surrounding the wound with circular motion (Fig. 53)
- **Important:** Never move a swab from the outside towards the wound again!

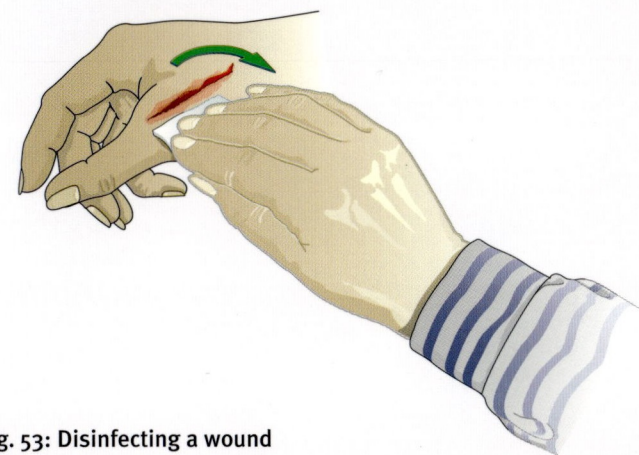

Fig. 53: Disinfecting a wound

> ⚠ An open wound always poses the risk of infection! In particular, tetanus germs are everywhere. Any wound can get infected and result in death. Always make sure that you are sufficiently protected against tetanus before starting your trip or voyage (Page 82).

Caring for larger wounds
⇘ Basic wound care
⇘ Stitching the wound
⇘ Agraffe band-aid

> ⚠ The advantage of stitching the wound is a secure closing of the wound. It is also likely to have better cosmetic results. Disadvantage: The need for materials—wound stitch, anesthesia, sterile utensils—and the requirements for training people to use local anesthesias, sterile materials, and medication are fairly high. There is also the danger of infection with untrained helpers. The closing of a wound with a stitch is, therefore, not recommended for novices. Alternatively, the agraffe band-aid can be used to close even-edged wounds (see Fig. 54).

Using an Agraffe Band-Aid
(*Note: Agraffe is a German term. A comparable brand would be Band-Aid® Tough-Strips® by Johnson & Johnson.)
⇘ Particularly suited to close flat-edged wounds, such as in cases of cutting injuries
⇘ **Important:** Some bandages stick less in case of humidity, greasy skin and hair—use alcoholic disinfectant, or possibly remove hair
⇘ Afterwards, place compress onto wound and affix with bandage or adhesive bandage
⇘ Daily change of dressing, leave off band-aid for now
⇘ In case of signs of infection (Page 19): Open wound and rinse

> **IMPORTANT**
>
> **Do not use Agraffe or other band-aids in case of...**
> • infected and bite wounds
> • wounds older than six hours
> • gaping wound edges
>
> In these cases, a wound must not be closed, only apply basic wound care!

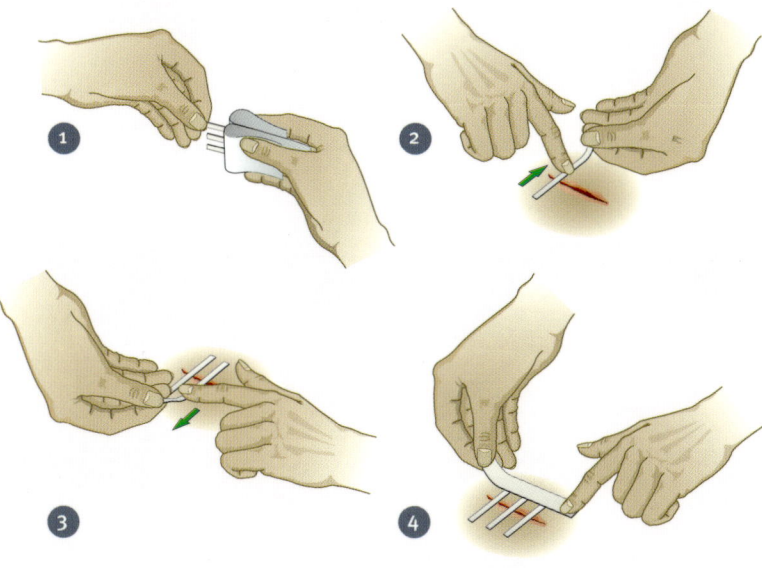

Fig. 54: Applying agraffe (or comparable) band-aid

❶ Clean hands. Take strips from the package.
❷ Apply strips with a distance of ca. 3 mm
❸ Apply strips
❹ Affix strips at their ends with adhesive tape

Medication Onboard

Disclaimer: The following recommendations are based on current scientific knowledge. Neither the author or the publisher is responsible for any misinformation.

> It is very important that you consult with your family doctor regarding possible pre-existing conditions that might make medications incompatible!

For crews up to about five people, one medical kit each is sufficient. For more people or longer trips, it is best to bring along several kits. The identification of the medication can be done using the number listed in the chart of the KV-COLUMN and may be helpful in case of a radio-assisted consultation.

Most of the medications should be able to be swallowed or be provided via a suppository. Some emergency medications (dexamethasone and adrenalin(e)), painkillers (s-ketamine and butyl scopolamine), and the blood thinner enoxaparin cannot be absorbed this way. In these cases, there needs to be a radio-assisted consultation to apply an injection into the muscle (intra-muscular) or under the skin (subcutaneous).

Necessary conditions:
- Provision with medication vials
- Familiarity with vials
- Familiarity with applying medications into the muscle or under the skin

> **IMPORTANT**
>
> Take advantage of radio-assisted consultations (Page 5). The independent use of prescription medication is only feasible when no other medical consultation is available. Always follow the instructions regarding dosage and side effects in the medication's package leaflet!

Legal Aspects (Liability)

Prescription medication has to be prescribed by a medical doctor. It may only be taken by the person for which it was prescribed. A prescription can occur while at sea during a radio-assisted consultation. If there is no prescription, a medication is not legally correct and might constitute personal injury. Giving medication can be life-saving; however, the risk of unwanted effects and legal liability must be taken into account. Problems may be averted by informing the patient about the planned treatment, maintaining a detailed protocol of the examination, as well as the intent to receive radio-assisted help

> **Categories for Medicines ...**
> Category 1: Standard equipment
> Category 2: For longer trips
> Category 3: Only bring with you if familiar with subcutaneous or intramuscular medication

Recommended Medication for the Journey (Chart)

No.	Active Substance	Brand Name (Example)	Cat.
	Gastrointestinal Diseases		
1	Charcoal	Kaopectate	1*
2	Elektrolyt-Glucose	Elotrans® (Pulver)	2
3	Loperamid	Imodium	2
4	Macrogol	Movicol® (Generic name: Polyethylene Glycol)	2
	Eye Inflammation and Injury		
5	Dexpanthenol	Bepanthen® (or any diaper rash creams)	1*
6	Tetryzolin	OptiClear, Tyzine (or Visine)	1
7	Gentamicin Sulfate	Refobacin® (5 ml or other eye-drop)	2
	Respiratory Illnesses		
8	Chlorhexidin	Chlorhexamed® (anti-septic)	1*
9	Benzocaine	Blistek® (or lozenges)	1*
10	Xylometazoline 0,1 %	Otrivin® (nasal drops)	1*
11	Ambroxol	Mucosolvan®	1
12	Codeine	Codipront® (drops or capsules)	2
	Aches and Pains		
13	Ibuprofen 400 mg	Ibudolor® (tablet)	1*
14	Paracetamol 500 mg	Benuron® (tablet)	1*
15	Metamizole	Novalgin®/Analgin (drops)	2
16	Tramadol	Tramal® (tablets)	1*
17	S-Ketamine 25 mg/ml	Ketanest® (liquid, 10 ml)	3
18	Butylscopolamine 20 mg	Buscopan® (tablet)	3

No. = serial number; Cat. = Category (see box on Page 67), * If more than five people are traveling or if it will be several days before you arrive at the next port, it is highly recommended that you pack several first aid kits; Rx. = medical prescription;

No.	Active Substance	Brand Name (Example)	Cat.
	Itching, itchiness		
19	Dimethindene maleate	Fenistil® (Gel)	1*
20	Prednicarbate	Prednitop®, Dermatop® (ointment)	2
21	Clotrimazole	Lotrimin® (ointment)	2
	Inflammation		
22	Povidone-iodine	Betadine® (Ointment, solution)	1*
23	Octenisept	Octenisept® (disinfectant solution)	1*
	Allergies		
24	Loratadine	Claritin® (also Zyrtec, Allegra, Benadryl)	2
25	Prednisolone 50 mg	Solu-Decortin® (Tablet)	2
26	Dexamethason 100 mg	Fortecortin® (already filled syringe)	3
27	Inhalers	Primatene® Mist (Atomizer)	2
28	Epinephrine (injection to the muscle)	EpiPen® (already filled syringe)	3
	Nausea, vomiting, seasickness		
29	Dimenhydrinate 20mg	Superpep® (chewing gum)	1*
30	Dimenhydrinate 50mg	Dramamine (suppository)	1*
31	Scopolamine	Scopoderm® (transdermal patch)	2*
32	Metoclopramide (Reglan)	Paspertin® (drip, uvula)	2
33	Metoclopramide (Reglan) 10 mg	Lasix® (capsule; used to help vomiting)	3
	For illnesses relating to children, see Page 77 and notes in text		
	Antibiotic		
34	Amoxicillin 500mg	Amoxy®, Amoxypen® (fluid, tablet)	1*
35	Amoxicillin/Clavulante 1 g	Ciprofloxacin® (tablet)	2
36	Ciprofloxacin 500 mg	Ciprobay® (Tablet)	2
37	Cotrimoxazole 960 mg	Bactrim, Septra, Sulfatrim (Tablet)	1
38	Metronidazole 400 mg	Clont® (Tablet)	2
39	Ceftriaxone 1 g	Rocephin® (injection)	3

No. = serial number; Cat. = Category (see box on Page 67), * If more than five people are traveling or if it will be several days before you arrive at the next port, it is highly recommended that you pack several first aid kits; Rx. = medical prescription;

No.	Active Substance	Brand Name (Example)	Cat.
	Emergency Medicines		
40	Diazepam	Valium® (Tablet or drip form)	2
41	Glyceryl trinitrate	Nitro-Spray®	2
42	Furosemide 20 mg	Furosemide® (Tablet, also Lasix)	2
43	Enoxaparin 100 mg/ml	Lovenox (10 ml solution)	3
44	Beclomethasone	Ventolair® (metered dose inhaler)	2
	Other Medicines		
45	Permethrin (synthetic insecticide)	NIX (solution against lice, scabies)	2
46	Lidocaine Hydrochloride (anesthetic)	Lidoject® sine 2 %® (glass capsule of local anesthesia)	3
47	Silver sulfadiazine	Flamazine® cream (to treat burns or skin infections)	2
48	Fettsalbe (fat ointment)	Linola® Fett (burn ointment cream)	1*
49	Pantoprazole	Protonix® (other options: Nexium, Prevacid, or Zantac)	2
50	Heilpflanzenöl (Medicinal plant oil)	Kamillosan® Ointment	1*
51	acetylsalicylic acid, aspirin	Ecotrin	2
52	Mebendazol 100 mg (Anti-worm powder)	Vermox® (Tablet)	2
53	Sodium hydrochloride 0,9 %	Infusion (500 ml)	3

No. = serial number; Cat. = Category (see box on Page 67), * If more than five people are traveling or if it will be several days before you arrive at the next port, it is highly recommended that you pack several first aid kits; Rx. = medical prescription;

> **TAKE NOTE**
>
> The medication in the following text refers to numbers that can be found in the Medication Chart (Pages 68-70).

Medication for Life-threatening Situations

- In case of Unconsciousness, Cardiac Arrest, or Profuse Bleeding: No options for medication applied by novices!
- In case of breathing difficulties after insect stings or bites or allergic reaction: In case of strong swelling: Cortizone, preferably 26, alternatively 44 or 25; Adrenaline (e.g. Epinephrine) preferably 28, alternatively or in addition 27
- In case of self-endangerment: Tranquilizer (40)

> In case of a known strong allergy to insect stings or bites, it is best to take preventive measures as to medication, e.g. taking along inhalers or a pre-filled syringe for intramuscular application (28). Note: It is very important that you learn how to apply the medication beforehand!

Medication with Guiding Symptom – Impaired Consciousness

- In case of Pain: Page 76
- In case of Fever: Fever-reducing medication 14; follow dosage (Page 76)!
- In case of Convulsion: Tranquilizer 40
- In case of Child's Fever Convulsion: Diazepam suppositories applied to the rectum
- In case of Psychiatric Illness with restlessness or aggression: Tranquilizer 40
- In case of Stiff Neck (meningismus) after an infection in the neck, throat, and mouth area: Antibiotic 39 (subcutaneous or intramuscular)
- In case of Impaired Consciousness:
  - Due to dehydration (e.g. diarrhea, vomiting): Page 73
  - In case of dehydration and deep unconsciousness (drinking not possible): Provide liquid as an infusion 53 (Page 80)
- In case of Impaired Consciousness and Very High Blood Pressure: High blood pressure can be the cause for impaired consciousness or a protective reaction of the brain; in no case should it be lowered to normal values.

> **IMPORTANT**
>
> - Diarrhea and vomiting can be life-threatening due to massive dehydration! In this case, sodium hydrocloride should be applied as an infusion (53, Page 80).
> - Extremely high blood pressure values, such as an upper blood pressure of over 200 mm Hg, should be lowered (emergency medication 41), but not under 160 mm Hg!

Medication with Guiding Symptoms – Impaired Breathing and Chest Pain

In case of infections of the breathing passages
- General measure: Drink a lot of fluids
- In case of a cold or indications for a middle ear infection (Page 25): Nose drops 10; inhaling oil 50
- In case of cough: Expectorant 11; in special cases cough medicine 12 (in case of painful dry cough)
- In case of bacterial infection of the breathing passages or pneumonia (Pages 25, 38): Antibiotic 34
- In case of bacterial tonsillitis (Page 25): Antibiotic 35
- In case of swallowing difficulties: Gargle solution 8; lozenges 9
- In case of pain: Page 76
- In case of pain when coughing or breathing deeply: Painkillers 13
- In case of breathing difficulties after rib fracture: 13-16, combine if necessary (Page 76)
- In case of fever: Fever-reducing medication 14; follow dosage instructions

> **IMPORTANT**
>
> After about three days of antibiotic medication—such as in the case of pneumonia—the patient's condition should improve; if it hasn't, call for a radio-assisted consultation!

In Case of Asthma and Bronchitis
- Continue with medication
- Cortisone 25 or 44; in case of strong breathing difficulties 26, anti-allergic 24, tranquilizer 40 (be careful with dosage!)
- In case of chronic bronchitis: Give antibiotic early, 34 or 35

In Cases of Heart and Circulation-related Illnesses
- In case of high blood pressure or diminished heart strength due to high blood pressure: Blood pressure medication 41
- In case of coronary syndrome, heart attack, pulmonary embolism, or obstructed blood vessel: tranquilizer 40
- In case of heart attack or high blood pressure: Increase urinary excretion (diuretic) 42
- In case of nausea and vomiting: 32 or 33
- In case of blood vessel obstruction: Blood thinner 43
- In case of heart attack: Blood thinner 43 and 51
- In case of heart attack, pulmonary embolism, or obstructed artery: Painkillers, see Page 76

In case of shock
- Due to allergic reaction: Cortison 25 or 26; Adrenaline 28
- Due to dehydration: Provide fluid as infusion 53 (Page 80)
- Due to diminished heart strength: See above (medication in case of heart and circulation problems)

> ⚠️
> - In case of indications for heart attack, pulmonary embolism, or obstructed artery: Never inject medication into a muscle!
> - Be careful when applying nitroglycerin (41) against high blood pressure: The decrease in blood pressure can be life-threatening; it is better to space out the applications than to apply in a single dose. Check blood pressure repeatedly after application.

Medication for Guiding Symptom – Abdominal Pain

- For all cases of abdominal pain: See Page 76
- In case of diarrhea, vomiting, and constipation without complications: Very sweet beverages, salty food, drink a lot of fluids, medical charcoal 1
- In case of dehydration (Page 19): Electrolyte concentrate 2
- In case of dehydration with impaired consciousness: Provide fluid as infusion 53 (Page 80)
- In case of more than about 10% of loss of body weight due to dehydration (about seven liters or 15 pints in case of an adult): Provide fluid via infusion 53 (life-threatening!)
- In case of diarrhea with blood (in the tropics, probable worm parasite infection): Vermicide 52
- To suppress diarrhea: 3
  Important: Only apply in special cases (e.g. while passing through a storm)!
- In case of vomiting: 30 or 32; in cases of serious vomiting, apply 33 as subcutaneous injection (Page 79)
- In case of constipation: drink a lot of fluids; if not sufficient, additionally 4
- In case of intestinal infection: Antibiotics are only rarely necessary; if they are in this case, 36
- In case of urinary tract infection and inflammation of the pelvis: Antibiotics 37
- In case of serious illnesses (appendicitis, gall bladder infection, intestinal obstruction): Always give antibiotics 35 and 38; provide fluid as infusion 53 (Page 80)

Medication in Case of Heat, Cold, or Water Emergencies

- In case of pain: Page 76
- In case of seizure due to sunstroke: 40
- In case of headaches due to sunstroke: 13 or 14
- In case of water inhalation due to drowning: Antibiotic 35
- In case of burns: Burn ointment or balm 47 or 48
- In case of burns with indication of wound infection: Antibiotic 35
- In case of breathing difficulties due to burns with smoke inhalation: Cortison 25, 26, or 44
- In case of any inhalation, large burns (more than 10% grade II or 5% grade III), large areas with frostbite (e.g. entire limb), and drowning accidents from stage II onwards without rapid improvement: Increase urine production 42 (to avoid pulmonary embolism and kidney damage) and stomach protection 49 (to avoid damage to the stomach mucosa)

Medication in Case of Injuries to the Locomotor System

- In case of pain: Page 76
- To prevent pain when changing posture: 17, in all cases combine with 40
- In case of nausea (also side effects of painkiller 16): 30 or 32
- In case of open fractures: Antibiotic 35
- To prevent thrombosis in case of immobilization after accident: Heparin as subcutaneous injection 43 (Page 79)
- In case of blood loss with shock (Page 41): Provide fluid via infusion 53 (Page 80)

Seasickness

Most affected are children between the ages of two and twelve. After the age of 50, the probability of seasickness decreases. Women are more affected than men. There is no real prophylaxis or medication against seasickness. In many cases, it is just a process of getting used to the movement of the vessel, after which the effects are diminished greatly or go away altogether.

Causes
Impairment of the balance system due to unusual movement and contradicting sensations.

How to recognize?
Starts with yawning and loss of appetite, followed by nausea, vomiting, vertigo, sweating, apathy; in severe cases, there can also be circulatory problems.

What can happen?
Self-endangerment and danger for crew and other passengers due to impaired vigilance and coordination problems. Seasick passengers or crew members often cannot participate in daily activities on board.

What to do?
Measures for preventing seasickness:
- Stable mental condition, get enough sleep, and avoid alcohol, nicotine, and eating heavy meals
- When on board, try to remain on deck and midships, observe the horizon towards the bow, avoid flexing or bending the upper body, participate in daily activities (take the helm)

Sometimes the following may be helpful:
- Acupuncture treatment before the voyage, acupressure wristbands, homeopathy
- Ginger (fresh or candies), Vitamin C (1 x per day 1 gr., as lozenges)
- Avoid food that is rich in histamines: e.g. salami, hard cheese, fresh tomatoes

How to handle a Seasick Person
- Observe, put on life-jacket or life belt
- Remain midships and observe the horizon
- In case of extended heavy vomiting: Watch for signs of dehydration (Page 19)
- Consider change of course or interrupting the trip

Medication:
There are no real efficient medication. Most medications have side-effects; primarily fatigue, but also depression and visual impairment. The medication should be taken before the start of the trip. Dimenhydrinate lozenges may be helpful once the seasickness sets in; also antihistamines (29, 30), anticholinergics (31), and dopamine antagonists (32, 33) as subcutaneous injections (Page 79).

Self-made replacement for electrolyte solution
Dissolve 1 teaspoon of salt, 8 teaspoons of sugar, and 1 pack of baking powder (if available) in 1 liter (2 pints) of water. Drink the solution during the day.

Medication for Other Injuries

Medication for Eye Problems
- In case of pain: Page 76
- In case of eye irritation: Eye balm or ointment 5; eye drops 6
- In case of eye infection: Add 7
- In case of foreign object in the eye: Anesthetize surface 46
- In case of eye injury: Tranquilizer 40; antibiotic 34

 Do not apply eye ointments in case of possible eye injury!

Medication for Toothaches and Infections of the Mouth and Throat Area
Causes: Accidents, tooth decay, defective denture
How to recognize? Pain, signs of infection at gums or mucous membranes (Page 19); damaged or loose fillings; irritated dental nerve: Short pain when irritated (cold, warm, sweet)

What to do?
- In case of irritated tooth nerve: Avoid irritation
- Bleeding (e.g. when losing a tooth) is stopped using compression such as with a sterile swab

An emergency dental kit is recommended to fix tooth damage (see Page 82)

Medication
- In case of toothache: Begin with 13; see Page 76
- In case of any tooth damage and infections of the mouth and throat areas: Keep good oral hygiene by rinsing several times a day and after every meal with 8, alternatively with 23, or warm saltwater solution
- In case of complicated infections of the mouth area: Antibiotics 34 or 35

Medication and Treatment for Itching
Causes: Usually insect stings or allergic reactions, sometimes fungal infection or contact with jellyfish
What to do? In case of contact with jellyfish, the following might be effective:
- Put on vinegar, rub with flour or shaving cream; after a few minutes remove carefully
- Warm water bath; 45ºC (113ºF) water temperature for 30-45 minutes.

- Careful with warm water baths: Danger of burns!
- Do not rinse the area with fresh water or alcohol!

Medication
- In case of itching after insect stings/bites and allergy: Antihistamine balm/ointment 19
- In case of itching skin eczemas and allergic reactions: Cortizone balm 20
- In case of itching fungal infection of skin and mucous membranes: Antimycotic (anti-fungal) balm 21

Medication and Treatment of Allergic Reactions
Causes: Typical allergic agents such as blooms and pollen, some medication (e.g. Penicillin), food (e.g. nuts), insect poisons
How to recognize? Reddening, itching, swelling, breathing difficulties (Page 14). Allergies may be limited to itching; however, there may be severe cases with circulatory collapse and shock (Page 41). It is common that an allergy is known as a pre-existing condition.
What to do? Remove from source, cool

Medication
- In case of light allergy: Antihistamine 24, Cortizone 25; in case of allergic cold 10
- In case of severe allergy (breathing difficulties!): Page 71

Medication for Care of Wounds
- In case of pain: Page 76
- In case of increased danger of infection (bite- or soiled/dirty wound): Disinfectant balm/ointment 22
- In case of wounds of hand or foot: Bathe in iodine solution 22
- In case of signs of infection (Page 19): Additional wound rinse with disinfectant 23, antibiotic 35
  Important: 22 and 23 can be given one after the other with time in between application; 23 needs to flow freely and must not be injected into closed wound openings.

> ⚠ Any infection can be life-threatening. Therefore, wounds need to be diligently cared for. If there is no improvement despite diligent care and taking antibiotics, it is imperative to request medical assistance (Page 5).

Medication to Treat Pain
Schematic for increasing pain intensities:
1. Paracetamol or NSAR or Metamizole
2. Paracetamol combined with NSAR or Metamizole
3. Paracetamol, NSAR, or Metamizole combined with light opiate (e.g. Tramadol)
4. Paracetamol, NSAR, Metamizole, or light Opiate combined with S-Ketamine/Diazepam

Paracetamol (14)
- e.g. Benuron®
- Beware: In case of liver diseases, during pregnancy; watch dosage for children due to danger of overdose (Page 77)!

Non-steroidal Anti-phlogistics (NSAR, 13)
- e.g. Ibuprofen®
- **Use:** In case of pain of articulation or inflammatory pain (e.g. bruised ribs, back pain, toothache)
- **Attention:** In case of impaired kidney function, stomach illness, weak heart, asthma, bronchitis; if taken for prolonged periods with known stomach problems, combine with gastric protection (e.g. Pantoprazole, 49)

Metamizole (15)
- e.g. Novalgin®
- **Use:** In case of pain affected by nerves (e.g. toothache); in case of abdominal pain
- Side effects: In rare cases, life-threatening side effects

> **IMPORTANT**
>
> Generally, the use of Novalgin is not be recommended!

Opiates (16)
- e.g. Amadol® capsules
- **Use:** In case of stronger pain
- Side effects: Fatigue
- **Attention:** In case of colic-like pain (e.g. urine or gall tract, pancreas), use Butylscopolamine (18)

S-Ketamine (17)
- e.g. Ketanest-S®
- **Use:** Strong painkiller, injected into a blood vessel, a muscle or under the skin. Advantage: protective reflexes and breathing are not affected if used correctly when compared to opiates
- Side effects: Possible hallucinations, therefore always combine with Diazepam (40)
- **Attention:** S-Ketamine requires a thorough instruction as to its application and dangers!

Others: Butylscopolamine (18)
- e.g. Buscopan®
- **Use:** In case of colic-like (wave-like) pain (e.g. gall stones or kidney stones)

Medication for Children
The choice depends on pre-existing illnesses and the geographic area. It is important to consult with a pediatrician before leaving! The basic equipment on board should consist of:
- Seasickness: Dimenhydrinate (e.g. Vomex® suppositories)
- Pains and fever: Acetaminophen (e.g. Benuron® as a liquid or suppositories); be sure to give the dosage according to the weight, as an overdose can be life-threatening!
- Fever convulsion: e.g. Diazepam (suppository)
- Cold and Sinus: Decongestant nasal spray or drops with concentration for children
- Cough: Ambroxol (e.g. Mucosolvan® as liquid)
- Barking cough, bronchitis, asthma, allergic reactions: Cortizone suppositories (e.g. Rectodelt®)

Dosage of Acetaminophen for children
Example:
- Body weight of the child: 30 kg / 65 lbs.
- Maximum dosage per day: 30 x 50 mg = 1500 mg
- Distributed across three daily dosages: 1500 : 3 = 500 mg per dose

A child with a weight of 30 kg / 65 lbs. therefore receives a maximum of 3 x 500 mg Acetaminophen per day.

Medication and Treatment for Infections – Antibiotics
Important areas of application are in italics.

> **PLEASE NOTE**
>
> Infections can be life-threatening if they are not treated. If you are unsure, or complications arise, or the treatment shows no improvement: take advantage of radio-assisted consultation (Page 5)!

Amoxicillin (34)
- **Form:** Tablets
- **Use:** Infections of the upper respiratory passages, infections of the tooth

Amoxicillin/Clavulanic Acid (35)
- **Form:** Tablets
- **Application:** Infections of the bone, articulation and skin; infection of the breathing passages and in the area of the middle ear (tonsils, outer auditory passage, para-nasal sinuses), bite wounds, important infections of the abdominal organs (e.g. peritonitis and appendicitis)

Ciprofloxacin (36)
- **Form:** Tablets
- **Use:** Gastrointestinal infections, gynecological and sexually transmissible diseases

Cotrimoxazol (37)
- **Form:** Tablets
- **Use:** Gall bladder infection (cystitis), pyelitis

Metronidazol (38)
- **Form:** Tablets
- **Use:** Infection of the abdominal organs, e.g. indications of appendicitis
- **Important:** Always provide in combination with another antibiotic (e.g. Amoxicillin/clavulanic acid, 35)

Medication for Emergencies

Diazepam (40)
- **Form:** Swallowed
- **Effect:** Supposed to prevent side effects from painkillers (17), such as hallucinations; tranquilizer
- **Use:** In addition to painkillers, as a tranquilizer (Page 72)

Glyceroltrinitrate (41)
- **Form:** Applied via a spray onto the mucus of the mouth (learn how to apply!)
- **Effect:** Lowers the blood pressure and widens the coronary arteries
- Side effects: Increases cardiac frequency
- **Use:** In case of high blood pressure, probably after heart attack or coronary syndrome (only after radio-assisted consultation!)

Furosemide (42)
- **Form:** Swallowed
- **Effect:** Increases urine production
- **Use:** In case of water accumulation in the lung (pulmonary edema) as a result of high blood pressure, heart weakness, or drowning accident

Enoxaparin (43)
- **Form:** Under the skin
- **Effect:** As a prevention against thrombosis in case of lack of movement (e.g. after a fracture) or after a heart attack and pulmonary edema
- **Use:** In case of fractures (see section starting on Page 55)

> **IMPORTANT**
>
> Bring along small syringes (1 ml)!

Beclomethasone (44)
- **Form:** Aerosol
- **Effect:** Widens the breathing passages
- **Use:** In case of smoke inhalation or strong allergic reaction

> **IMPORTANT**
>
> The application of Beclomethasone can be difficult – follow instructions closely!

Ceftriaxone (39)
- **Form:** Injection (deep intramuscular, into the buttocks, in exceptional cases also under the skin), because the oral antibiotics are not sufficiently effective; very expensive
- **Use:** Meningitis, wide-ranging antibiotic for many infections (e.g. breathing passages, ear, nose, and throat (ENT) and urologic area, bones, skin)

 The application of Ceftriaxone requires knowledge about administering medication into a muscle!

Medication – Injection

If medication cannot be swallowed or administered as a suppository, an injection will be necessary, meaning giving the medication via a syringe.

 Giving an injection is a potentially dangerous procedure.

Options
There are three methods for injections:
- Subcutaneous, into the fat layer under the skin
- Intramuscular, into a muscle
- Intravenous, into a vein

The subcutaneous injection is the most simple method and has the smallest risk of infection. Medical novices can perform it after some training. The disadvantage is that the medication is absorbed more slowly than an intramuscular or intravenous injection.

Supplies
- Vials, syringe, 2 cannules (for the injection)
- Disinfectant, swab, band-aid
- Examination gloves

Sometimes pre-filled syringes are available, e.g. for adrenaline and Cortizone; in many cases, however, the medication needs to be drawn from a vial (Fig. 55).

How to do? – Preparing the Injection
- Take vial: Check the name and storage and expiration date
- Break off the empty neck of the vial (1): Hold neck between thumb and index finger, place the thumb at the dotted mark, and break off the neck towards the back (**Attention: risk of injury!**)
- Place sterile cannule with protective cap onto the syringe (2)
- Remove protective cap, insert cannule into the vial, and draw medication (3)
- Keep it clean: Do not touch cannule at its tip and do not put down without its protective cap!
- Put protective cap onto the cannule, remove cannule
- Put injection cannule with protective cap onto the syringe, remove protective cap
- Remove air from the syringe: Hold cannule vertically and press out air (4)

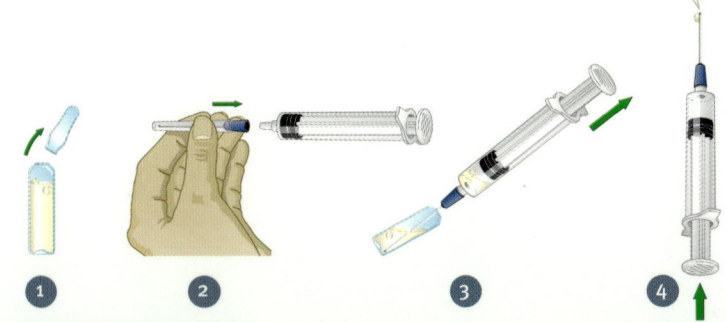

Fig. 55: Handling vials

How to do? – Giving the Injection
↘ Watch hygiene: Wash and disinfect hands, wear examination gloves, disinfect punctured area
↘ Choose area without swelling or inflammation (thigh, abdomen, upper arms, Fig. 56); lift a fold of skin with one hand and quickly insert needle at an angle of about 15 degrees, the entire needle
↘ Did you catch a blood vessel? Pull at the syringe to test. If blood appears, push forward or pull back cannule and check again
↘ Inject medication
↘ Remove cannule, cover punctured area with band-aid
↘ Observe patient: Any effect will take at least 10 minutes

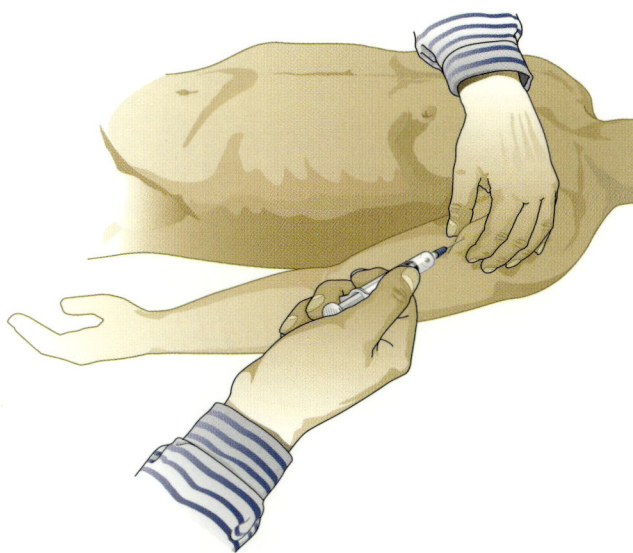

Fig. 56: Injection – Medicine given under the skin (subcutaneous)

What can happen?
↘ Helper gets injured opening the vial
↘ Inflammation of the punctured area
↘ Allergic reaction

Medication or Fluid Application – Infusion
Severe dehydration—for example in case of fever, diarrhea, vomiting, or impaired consciousness—can be life-threatening. However, the affected person may often not be able to drink. In cases where 10 percent of the body weight (about 7 liters / 15 pints in case of adults) has been lost or in cases of dehydration with impaired consciousness (Page 35), fluid should be applied via an infusion.

 Infusions are potentially dangerous!

Options
There are three options to provide fluid:
↘ Subcutaneous, into the fat layer under the skin
↘ Intravenous, into a vein
↘ Using a feeding tube
  Puncturing a vein and inserting a feeding tube can be challenging. However, subcutaneous infusions can be performed by novices after some training (Fig. 57).

Supplies
↘ Infusion fluid (e.g. 500 ml plastic bottles with sodium hydrocloride solution 0.9%)
↘ Infusion tube (infusion system); can be used for several successive infusions
↘ Cannule or venous access
↘ Disinfectant, swab, band-aid
↘ Examination gloves

TIP When puncturing the skin, use a so-called "venous access": a flexible plastic tube is all that remains and poses no risk of injury. Recommended sizes for the venous access: pink (diameter 1.2 mm) or green (diameter 1.4 mm).

How to do? – Preparing the Infusion
- Check appropriate storage and expiration dates of the materials and the medication
- Prepare infusion bottle: Remove protective ring at the neck
- Close infusion system: Move wheel to the bottom (1a), press spur into the opening of the infusion bottle's neck (1c)
- Fill drip chamber (1b): Place bottle with the neck towards the bottom and fill the drip chamber by pressing repeatedly — **Attention:** Only fill about 50%!
- Fill system: Move wheel to the top; the drip chamber receives drops. Close infusion system in case fluid leaks from the system

How to do? – Giving the Infusion
- Choose puncture area: Abdomen or thigh (2)
- Prepare puncture: See subcutaneous injection (Page 80)
- After the puncture, remove the steel cannula (3) of the venous access and tape the part remaining under the skin; attach well
- Connect the infusion system with a twisting push: Place the bottle as high as possible above the patient and attach (e.g. attach to the handrail)
- Carefully open the system and control drip frequency: About 1 drop / second

What can happen?
- Burning pain at the beginning of the infusion
- Inflammation of the punctured area

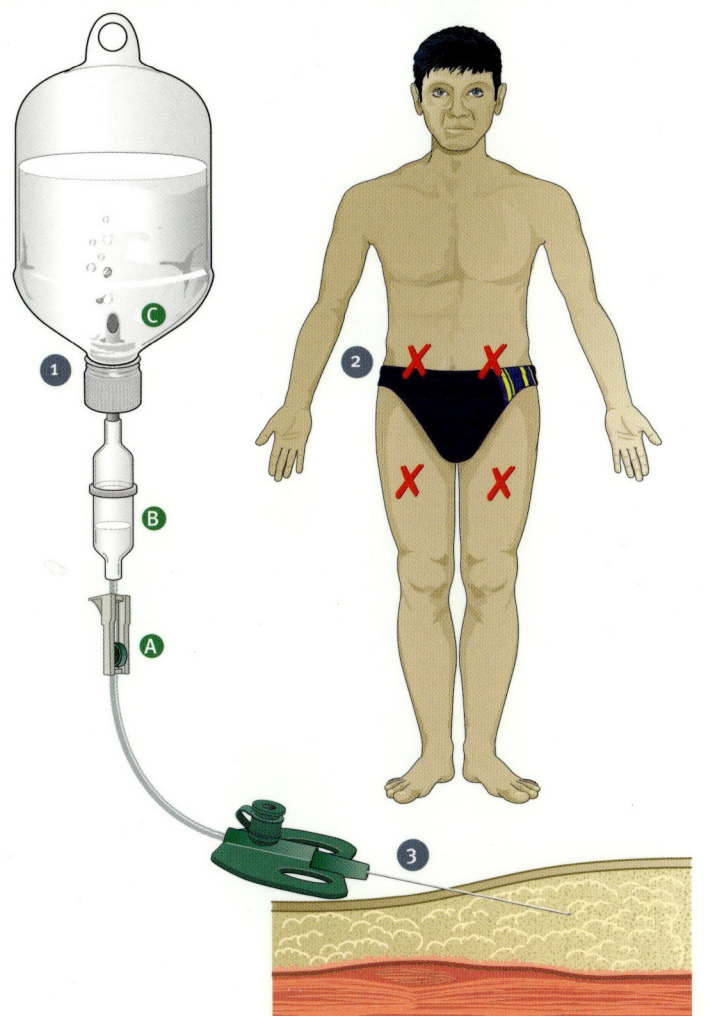

Fig. 57: Infusion – Fluid infusion under the skin (subcutaneous)

❶ Infusion bottle with infusion system: a=wheel, b=drip chamber, c=spur
❷ Best puncture areas for the infusion
❸ Venous access, under the skin (subcutaneous)

Appendix

Forms and Questionnaires
The comprehensive forms and additional questionnaires can be obtained at www.seadoc.de (in German and English)

Medical Information
Each passenger should provide information regarding his medical condition prior to a trip. This information can be very important for helpers in case of an emergency and should be kept in an envelope by the captain.
- Personal information: name, age, height, weight
- Adresses and telephone numbers of relatives and family doctor
- Basic parameters while at rest: blood pressure and pulse
- Prior illnesses, diseases, operations and allergies
- Use of medication, time of application and place of storage

Examination
Make annotations while performing the examination:
- General: Time of examination, patient's name, age, height, and weight
- Illness: Main problem, start of illness, slow or fast onset, previous problem? If so, what was the treatment?
- Consciousness: Alertness, orientation, speech, strength, sensitivity
- Breathing: Frequency, breathing difficulties, prolonged exhalation phase, pain while inhaling
- Circulation: Pulse, blood pressure, heart frequency, chest pain, signs for diminished cardiac strength
- Abdomen: Existing warning signs? Which? Noticeable stool or urine changes
- Skin: Color, humidity, any indication of dehydration
- Pain: Where, since when, how (blunt, bright, wave-shaped), increasing intensity?
- Injuries: Where, what, how, wrong position?
- Burn: Where, how, size, grade of burns, signs of smoke inhalation? Pain?
- Other: Body temperature, additional observations

Radio-assisted consultation
A radio-assisted consultation will provide valuable information and results if it is well-prepared.

General Information
- Who is calling, name of ship and call sign, current position, and closest port
- How many persons are affected, threat to life?

Information about the patient:
- Name, age, weight, important prior illnesses
- Main problem? Prior appearance? Onset of illness? Cause or trigger?
- Treatment so far, medication
- Suspected diagnosis

Basic findings:
- Attention, blood pressure, pulse, rate of breath, body temperature, skin color, abdomen

Various:
- Keep the medications of the patient and a list of the medications available on board handy

Protocol
Take note of the basic findings at regular intervals, e.g. every three hours with stable patients, every ten minutes in critical situation.
- Pulse, blood pressure, breathing rate, temperature
- Attention, strength
- Applied medication

Vaccines
Are you planning a longer trip? Have a look at the vaccination card. Health care insurance usually does not cover the vaccination for travel purposes, however, some vaccinations are recommended when traveling to risk areas. Other vaccines depend on the recommendation, your particular trip, and the type and length of the trip. Take advantage of consultation services or tropical institutes and vaccination centers.

As an adult you should be vaccinated against the following diseases and illnesses:
- Tetanus: Refresh every 10 years
- Diphteria: Refresh every 10 years

You should be vaccinated against the following diseases if you are over 60 or if your lung is damaged (chronic bronchitis, asthma, smoking):
- Pneumococci: Refresh every 6 years
- Influenza: Every year around August/September

If you plan a longer trip, the following vaccines are recommended depending on your destination and the type of journey:
- ESME: Early Summer Meningoencephalitis
- Hepatitis A and B
- Typhus
- Polio
- Yellow fever

Courses and Information
- Red Cross, www.redcross.org

Commercial Sources
- Equipment and medication is available at most local pharmacies
- Complete sets and defibrillators can be purchased at Seadoc, www.seadoc.de, or Ocean Medical www.oceanmedicalinternational.com

Contents

Introduction	2
Before the Trip	**3**
The Emergency Call	5
Life-threatening Situations	**6**
Unconsciousness	7
Massive Bleeding	13
Severe Breathing Difficulties	14
Self-endangerment due to Impaired Consciousness	17
The Examination	**18**
Standard Values	18
Examination Methods	19
Examination of Consciousness and Nervous System	20
Examination of Breathing Passages, Breath, Heart and Circulation	22
Examination of Abdomen	27
Body Check after an Accident	30
Guiding Symptoms and Illnesses	**31**
Guiding Symptom – Impaired Consciousness	33
Illnesses and Diseases with Impaired Consciousness	34
Guiding Symptoms – Breathing Difficulties and Chest Pains	36
Illnesses and Diseases of the Lung, Breathing Passages, Heart, and Circulatory System	38
Guiding Symptom – Abdominal Pain	44
Stomach Illness	45
Effects of Heat, Cold, or Water	**48**
Hypothermia	49
Frostbite	50
Burn Wounds	51
Injuries of the Locomotor System	**54**
How to recognize	55
What can happen?	56
What to do after an Accident	56
Special characteristics in case of Sprains and Fractures	56
Change of Position	56
Stabilization and Immobilization	58
Taking care of Open Fractures	61
Other Injuries	**62**
Eye Irritation and Inflammation	62
Foreign Object in Eye	62
Eye Injury	62
Nosebleed	63
Hematoma under the Finger- or Toenail	63
Fishhook injury	63
Wound Care	**64**
Medication Onboard	**67**
Recommended Medication for the Journey (Chart)	68
Seasickness	74
Medication for Other Injuries	75
Medication – Injection	79
Medication or Fluid Application – Infusion	80
Appendix	**82**

US $24.99

ISBN: 978-0-87033-636-2

Medical emergencies can happen anytime and anywhere, so first aid training can be very useful. It can be especially important if you are out at sea, where medical assistance can be hours or even days away. When onboard a seagoing vessel, even minor accidents, such as burns, sprains, and fractures, have the potential to become life-threatening. Being prepared and knowing essential first aid care can be the difference between life and death. This illustrated instructional guide offers a quick overview for the correct way to provide first aid. Chapters include standard medical examinations, different illnesses and related symptoms, effects of heat, cold, and water, and collecting relevant information about a sick or injured person. Such information is valuable not only for the person providing first aid, but also to give over the radio, because it may facilitate the decision-making about treatment strategy, thus saving lives under extreme circumstances.